✔ KU-202-450

Nursing Calculations

SEVENTH EDITION

J. D. Gatford
Mathematics Teacher, Melbourne, Australia

N. Phillips
DipAppSci(Nsg) BN GDipAdvNsg(Educ) MNS
Lecturer, School of Nursing and Midwifery, La Trobe University,
Bundoora, Australia

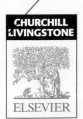

CHURCHILL
LIVINGSTONE

ELSEVIER

Edinburgh London New York Oxford Philadelphia St Louis Sydney Toronto 2006

CHURCHILL LIVINGSTONE

ELSEVIER

An imprint of Elsevier Limited

First edition 1982
Second edition 1987
Third edition 1990
Fourth edition 1994

Fifth edition 1998
Sixth edition 2002
Seventh edition 2006
Reprinted 2007 (twice), 2008

ISBN: 978 0 443 10288 2

British Library Cataloguing in Publication Data
A catalogue record for this book is available from the British Library

Library of Congress Cataloguing in Publication Data
A catalogue record for this book is available from the Library of Congress

Note
Neither the Publisher nor the authors assume any responsibility for any loss or injury and/or damage to persons or property arising out of or related to any use of the material contained in this book. It is the responsibility of the treating practitioner, relying on independent expertise and knowledge of the patient, to determine the best treatment and method of application for the patient.

The Publisher

ELSEVIER your source for books, journals and multimedia in the health sciences

www.elsevierhealth.com

Working together to grow libraries in developing countries

www.elsevier.com | www.bookaid.org | www.sabre.org

ELSEVIER   BOOK AID International   Sabre Foundation

The publisher's policy is to use **paper manufactured from sustainable forests**

Printed in China

Contents

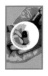

Preface to the Seventh Edition

This edition contains additional material suggested by nurse educators. The continuing positive feedback on our well-established book, from *all* sections of the nursing profession, is greatly appreciated and most encouraging.

An exercise using proprietary labels from drug containers has been added to the chapter on dosages for oral medication and also to the chapter on drug dosages for injection.

Paediatric calculations are now consolidated into one chapter.

Colour has been introduced to further improve the appearance of the book and to highlight key parts of the text.

Drug dosages have again been revised and updated throughout the text. However, it must be noted that the aim of *Nursing Calculations* is to teach relevant skills in *arithmetic*. The book is *not* meant to be used as a pharmacology reference.

J.D.G., N.P.
Melbourne 2006

Preface to the First Edition

This book was written at the request of nurse educators and with considerable help from them. It deals with elements of the arithmetic of nursing, especially the arithmetic of basic pharmacology.

The book begins with a diagnostic test which is carefully related to a set of review exercises in basic arithmetic. Answers to the test are supplied at the back of the book, and are keyed to the corresponding review exercises.

Students should work through those exercises which correspond to errors in the diagnostic test. The other exercises may also, of course, be worked through to improve speed and accuracy.

Throughout the other chapters of the book there are adequate, well graded exercises and problems. Each chapter includes several worked examples. Answers are given to all questions.

Suggestions and comments from nurse educators and students on the scope and content of this book would be welcomed. The hope is that its relevance to nursing needs will be maintained in subsequent editions.

J.D.G.
Melbourne 1982

Acknowledgements

The authors would like to thank those nurse educators, nurses and pharmacists who provided advice and constructive criticism during the preparation of this seventh edition.

The authors wish also to thank Ninette Premdas, Senior Commissioning Editor, who recommended a seventh edition; Katrina Mather, Development Editor, who managed the project; Tonks Fawcett of the Department of Nursing Studies at Edinburgh University; Theo Kossart, from the Intensive Care Unit of The Alfred Hospital; Meg Bayley, Diabetic Educator, Melbourne; Gavin Hawkins, for computer graphics; and Hannah Mason of the sanofi-aventis Group.

We are grateful to the sanofi-aventis Group and to GlaxoSmithKline Australia Pty Ltd for permission to reproduce drug labels for inclusion in this book.

John Gatford wishes to thank his wife, Elaine, for related secretarial work and for her continued patience and understanding during the course of this ongoing project.

1. A review of basic calculations

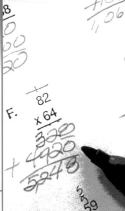

In this chapter, a list of mathematical terms is followed by a diagnostic test. This test is designed to pinpoint those areas of your arithmetic which need revising before you commence nursing calculations.

Attempt all questions.

Answers are supplied at the back of the book, and direct you to particular exercises, according to the *errors* in your test answers.

For example, if you make an error in answering either question 1 or question 2, then you will be asked to do *Exercise 1A*. Or, if your answer to question 3 or 4 is wrong, you should do *Exercise 1B*.

Remember that this test is designed to *help* you.

CHAPTER CONTENTS

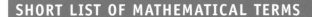

SHORT LIST OF MATHEMATICAL TERMS

Whole numbers

Whole number:
A number without fractions.

e.g. 5, 17, 438, 10 592.

Whole numbers are also known as *integers.*

Fractions

The full name for a fraction such as $\frac{1}{4}$ is *vulgar fraction.*

However, the name **fraction** is used in this book, for simplicity.

e.g. $\frac{3}{8}$ $\frac{17}{5}$ $\frac{1}{6}$ $\frac{9}{4000}$

Numerator:
The top number in a fraction.
e.g. In the fraction $\frac{3}{8}$ the numerator is 3.

Denominator:
The bottom number in a fraction.
e.g. In the fraction $\frac{3}{8}$ the denominator is 8.

Proper and improper fractions

A *proper* fraction is a fraction in which the numerator is *smaller* than the denominator.

e.g. $\frac{1}{4}$ $\frac{5}{8}$ $\frac{11}{100}$

An *improper* fraction is a fraction in which the numerator is *larger* than the denominator.

e.g. $\frac{5}{3}$ $\frac{32}{7}$ $\frac{100}{9}$

An improper fraction can be converted to a mixed number.

e.g. $\frac{5}{3} = 1\frac{2}{3}$ $\frac{32}{7} = 4\frac{4}{7}$ $\frac{100}{9} = 11\frac{1}{9}$

Mixed number:
Partly a whole number, partly a fraction.

e.g. $1\frac{5}{8}$ $4\frac{1}{2}$ $10\frac{4}{5}$

A mixed number can be converted to an improper fraction.

e.g. $1\frac{5}{8} = \frac{13}{8}$ $4\frac{1}{2} = \frac{9}{2}$ $10\frac{4}{5} = \frac{54}{5}$

Decimals

Decimal:
Generally used to mean a number that includes a decimal point.
e.g. 6.35, 0.748, 0.002, 236.5

Decimal places:
Numbers to the right of the decimal point.

e.g. 6.35 has 2 decimal places.
     0.748 has 3 decimal places.
     0.002 has 3 decimal places.
     236.5 has 1 decimal place.

Place value (in decimals):
To the right of the decimal point are tenths, hundredths, thousandths, etc...
e.g. In the number 0.962, there are 9 tenths, 6 hundredths and 2 thousandths.

Percentages

Percentage:
Number of parts per hundred parts.
e.g. 14% means 14 parts per 100 parts.
     2.5% means 2.5 parts per 100 parts.

A percentage may be less than 1%.

e.g. 0.3% = 0.3 parts per 100 = 3 parts per 1000
     0.04% = 0.04 parts per 100 = 4 parts per 10 000

Other terms

Divisor:
The number by which you are dividing.
e.g. In the division $495 \div 15$, the divisor is 15.

Factors:
When a number is divided by one of its **factors**, the answer is a whole number (i.e. there is no remainder).
e.g. The factors of 12 are 1, 2, 3, 4, 6 and 12.
     The factors of 20 are 1, 2, 4, 5, 10 and 20.
     The number 1 is a factor of *every* number.

Common factors:
Two different numbers may have **common factors**; factors which are *common* to both numbers.
e.g. 1, 2 and 4 are the common factors of 12 and 20.

Simplify:
Write as simply as possible.

Calculate the value of:
The answer will be a number.

DIAGNOSTIC TEST

1 *Multiply*

  a 83×10 **b** 83×100 **c** 83×1000

2 *Multiply*

  a 0.0258×10 **b** 0.0258×100 **c** 0.0258×1000

3 *Divide. Write answers as decimals.*

  a $3.78 \div 10$ **b** $3.78 \div 100$ **c** $3.78 \div 1000$

4 *Divide. Write answers as decimals.*

  a $\dfrac{569}{10}$ **b** $\dfrac{569}{100}$ **c** $\dfrac{569}{1000}$

5 *Complete*

  a *1 kilogram = ... grams*

  b *1 gram = ... milligrams*

  c *1 milligram = ... micrograms*

  d *1 litre = ... millilitres*

Write answers to 6, 7, 8 and 9 in decimal form.

6 a *Change 0.83 kg to grams.*

  b *Change 6400 g to kilograms.*

7 a *Change 0.78 grams to milligrams.*

  b *Change 34 milligrams to grams.*

8 a *Change 0.086 milligrams to micrograms.*

  b *Change 294 micrograms to milligrams.*

9 a *Change 2.4 litres to millilitres.*

  b *Change 965 millilitres to litres.*

10 a *Change 0.07 L to mL.*

  b *Change 0.007 L to mL.*

  c *Which is larger: 0.07 L or 0.007 L?*

11 a *Convert 0.045 g to mg*

  b *Convert 0.45 g to mg.*

  c *Which is heavier: 0.045 g or 0.45 g?*

12 *Multiply*

  a 9×3 **b** 0.9×3

  c 0.9×0.3 **d** 0.09×0.03

13 *Multiply*

  a 78×6 **b** 7.8×0.6

  c 0.78×6 **d** 7.8×0.06

14 *Which of the numbers 2, 3, 4, 5, 6, 10, 12 are* **factors** *of 48?*

15 *Which of the numbers 2, 3, 5, 6, 7, 9, 11 are* **factors** *of 126?*

16 *Simplify ('cancel down')*

  a $\dfrac{16}{24}$ **b** $\dfrac{56}{72}$

17 *Simplify*

  a $\dfrac{45}{600}$ **b** $\dfrac{175}{400}$

18 *Simplify*

  a $\dfrac{40}{50}$ **b** $\dfrac{60}{90}$ **c** $\dfrac{90}{150}$

19 *Simplify*

  a $\dfrac{350}{500}$ **b** $\dfrac{1200}{1500}$ **c** $\dfrac{1600}{4000}$

20 *Simplify ('cancel down'). Leave answers as improper fractions.*

  a $\dfrac{65}{20}$ **b** $\dfrac{275}{50}$ **c** $\dfrac{500}{80}$

21 *Simplify ('cancel down'). Leave answers as improper fractions.*

  a $\dfrac{700}{120}$ **b** $\dfrac{400}{125}$ **c** $\dfrac{600}{250}$

22 *Simplify. Leave answers as improper fractions, where these occur.*

  a $\dfrac{0.6}{0.9}$ **b** $\dfrac{0.45}{0.5}$ **c** $\dfrac{200}{4.5}$ **d** $\dfrac{0.09}{0.05}$

23 *Round-off each number correct to* **one** *decimal place.*

  a 0.68   **b** 1.82   **c** 0.35

24 *Write each number correct to* **two** *decimal places.*

  a 0.374   **b** 2.625   **c** 0.516

25 *Write each number correct to* **three** *decimal places.*

  a 1.6081   **b** 0.5698   **c** 2.6565

26 *Change to exact decimal equivalents.*

  a $\dfrac{5}{8}$ **b** $\dfrac{9}{20}$ **c** $\dfrac{17}{25}$ **d** $\dfrac{31}{40}$

27 *Change to decimals correct to* **one** *decimal place.*

  a $\dfrac{1}{6}$ **b** $\dfrac{3}{7}$ **c** $\dfrac{7}{9}$

28 *Change to decimals correct to* **two** *decimal places.*

  a $\dfrac{5}{7}$ **b** $\dfrac{5}{9}$

29 *Change to decimals correct to* **three** *decimal places.*

  a $\dfrac{7}{30}$ **b** $\dfrac{59}{70}$

Check your answers on p 117–118

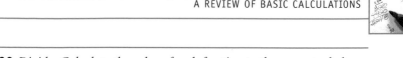

30 *Divide. Calculate the value of each fraction to the nearest whole number.*

  a $\dfrac{95}{3}$ **b** $\dfrac{225}{4}$

31 *Divide. Calculate the value of each fraction correct to one decimal place.*

  a $\dfrac{55}{6}$ **b** $\dfrac{65}{9}$

32 *Change to mixed numbers.*

  a $\dfrac{17}{2}$ **b** $\dfrac{67}{3}$ **c** $\dfrac{113}{5}$

33 *Change to improper fractions.*

  a $2\frac{3}{4}$ **b** $12\frac{5}{6}$ **c** $28\frac{2}{5}$

34 *Multiply. Simplify where possible.*

  a $\dfrac{2}{3} \times \dfrac{5}{6}$ **b** $\dfrac{5}{8} \times \dfrac{12}{7}$ **c** $\dfrac{9}{10} \times \dfrac{4}{9}$

MULTIPLICATION BY 10, 100 AND 1000

The examples show two methods of multiplying by 10, 100 and 1000, a long method and a short method. The short method is recommended.

Examples

i 0.36 × 10   **ii** 0.36 × 100   **iii** 0.36 × 1000

Long method

i	0.36	**ii**	0.36	**iii**	0.36
	× 10		× 100		× 1000
	3.60		36.00		360.00

All of these answers can be simplified: 3.60 = 3.6, 36.00 = 36, 360.0 = 360

Short method

i 0.36 × 10   = 3.6   = 3.6
ii 0.36 × 100   = 36.   = 36
iii 0.36 × 1000 = 360. = 360

Notes
• Use zeros to make up places, where necessary.
• If the answer is a whole number, the decimal point may be omitted.

Summary of short method

To multiply by	Move the decimal point
10	1 place right
100	2 places right
1000	3 places right

Exercise 1A   *Multiply*

1 0.68×10
0.68×100
0.68×1000

2 0.975×10
0.975×100
0.975×1000

3 3.7×10
3.7×100
3.7×1000

4 5.62×10
5.62×100
5.62×1000

5 77×10
77×100
77×1000

6 825×10
825×100
825×1000

7 0.2×10
0.2×100
0.2×1000

8 0.046×10
0.046×100
0.046×1000

9 0.0147×10
0.0147×100
0.0147×1000

10 0.006×10
0.006×100
0.006×1000

11 3.76×10
3.76×100
3.76×1000

12 0.639×10
0.639×100
0.639×1000

13 0.075×10
0.075×100
0.075×1000

14 0.08×10
0.08×100
0.08×1000

15 0.003×10
0.003×100
0.003×1000

16 0.0505×10
0.0505×100
0.0505×1000

Check your answers on p 119

DIVISION BY 10, 100 AND 1000

Example A *Short method*

i	$37.8 \div 10$	i	$37.8 \div 10 \quad = 3.\overset{\frown}{7}8$
ii	$37.8 \div 100$	ii	$37.8 \div 100 \quad = 0.\overset{\frown}{3}78$
iii	$37.8 \div 1000$	iii	$37.8 \div 1000 = 0.\overset{\frown}{0}378$

Notes
- Use zeros to make up places, where necessary.
- For numbers less than one, write a zero before the decimal point.

Example B

A division may be written as a fraction.

Evaluate   i $\dfrac{0.984}{10}$ i $\dfrac{0.984}{10} = 0.0984$

     ii $\dfrac{0.984}{100}$ ii $\dfrac{0.984}{100} = 0.00984$

    iii $\dfrac{0.984}{1000}$ iii $\dfrac{0.984}{1000} = 0.000984$

Summary of short method

To divide by	Move the decimal point
10	1 place left
100	2 places left
1000	3 places left

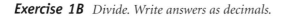

Exercise 1B *Divide. Write answers as decimals.*

1 $98.4 \div 10$
$98.4 \div 100$
$98.4 \div 1000$

2 $5.91 \div 10$
$5.91 \div 100$
$5.91 \div 1000$

3 $2.6 \div 10$
$2.6 \div 100$
$2.6 \div 1000$

4 $307 \div 10$
$307 \div 100$
$307 \div 1000$

5 $82 \div 10$
$82 \div 100$
$82 \div 1000$

6 $7 \div 10$
$7 \div 100$
$7 \div 1000$

7 $3 \div 10$
$3 \div 100$
$3 \div 1000$

8 $7.5 \div 10$
$7.5 \div 100$
$7.5 \div 1000$

9 $\dfrac{68}{10}$

$\dfrac{68}{100}$

$\dfrac{68}{1000}$

10 $\dfrac{2.29}{10}$

$\dfrac{2.29}{100}$

$\dfrac{2.29}{1000}$

11 $\dfrac{51.4}{10}$

$\dfrac{51.4}{100}$

$\dfrac{51.4}{1000}$

12 $\dfrac{916}{10}$

$\dfrac{916}{100}$

$\dfrac{916}{1000}$

13 $\dfrac{67.2}{10}$

$\dfrac{67.2}{100}$

$\dfrac{67.2}{1000}$

14 $\dfrac{387}{10}$

$\dfrac{387}{100}$

$\dfrac{387}{1000}$

15 $\dfrac{8.94}{10}$

$\dfrac{8.94}{100}$

$\dfrac{8.94}{1000}$

16 $\dfrac{0.707}{10}$

$\dfrac{0.707}{100}$

$\dfrac{0.707}{1000}$

Check your answers on p 119

CONVERTING METRIC UNITS

Memorise

> 1 kilogram (kg) = 1000 grams (g)
> 1 gram (g) = 1000 milligrams (mg)
> 1 milligram (mg) = 1000 micrograms (mcg)
> 1 litre (L) = 1000 millilitres (mL)

Note

There are two symbols in use for microgram: μg and mcg. You may see both of these symbols used on drug charts. Doctors and nurses now more commonly use mcg.

Example A *Change 0.6 kg to grams.*

$$0.6 \text{ kg} = 0.6 \times 1000 \text{ g}$$
$$= 600 \text{ g}$$

Example B *Change 375 g to kilograms.*

$$375 \text{ g} = 375 \div 1000 \text{ kg}$$
$$= 0.375 \text{ kg}$$

Example C *Change 0.67 g to milligrams.*

$$0.67 \text{ g} = 0.67 \times 1000 \text{ mg}$$
$$= 670 \text{ mg}$$

Example D *Change 23 mg to grams.*

$$23 \text{ mg} = 23 \div 1000 \text{ g}$$
$$= 0.023 \text{ g}$$

Example E *Change 0.075 mg to micrograms.*

$$0.075 \text{ mg} = 0.075 \times 1000 \text{ mcg}$$
$$= 75 \text{ mcg}$$

Example F *Change 185 mcg to milligrams.*

$$185 \text{ mcg} = 185 \div 1000 \text{ mg}$$
$$= 0.185 \text{ mg}$$

Example G *Change 1.3 L to millilitres.*

$$1.3 \text{ L} = 1.3 \times 1000 \text{ mL}$$
$$= 1300 \text{ mL}$$

Example H *Change 850 mL to litres.*

$$850 \text{ mL} = 850 \div 1000 \text{ L}$$
$$= 0.85 \text{ L}$$

Exercise 1C *Write all answers in decimal form.*

Change to grams.
1 5 kg   **2** 2.4 kg   **3** 0.75 kg   **4** 1.625 kg

Change to kilograms.
5 7000 g   **6** 935 g   **7** 85 g   **8** 3 g

Change to milligrams.
9 4 g   **11** 0.69 g   **13** 0.035 g   **15** 0.655 g
10 8.7 g   **12** 0.02 g   **14** 0.006 g   **16** 4.28 g

Change to grams.
17 6000 mg   **19** 865 mg   **21** 70 mg   **23** 5 mg
18 7250 mg   **20** 95 mg   **22** 2 mg   **24** 125 mg

Change to micrograms.
25 0.195 mg   **28** 0.075 mg   **31** 0.625 mg
26 0.6 mg   **29** 0.08 mg   **32** 0.098 mg
27 0.75 mg   **30** 0.001 mg

Change to milligrams.
33 825 mcg   **37** 10 mcg
34 750 mcg   **38** 5 mcg
35 65 mcg   **39** 200 mcg
36 95 mcg   **40** 30 mcg

Change to millilitres.
41 2 L   **44** $4\frac{1}{2}$ L   **47** 0.8 L
42 30 L   **45** 1.6 L   **48** 0.75 L
43 $1\frac{1}{2}$ L   **46** 2.24 L

Change to litres.
49 4000 mL   **51** 625 mL   **53** 95 mL   **55** 5 mL
50 10 000 mL   **52** 350 mL   **54** 60 mL   **56** 2 mL

Check your answers on p 119–120

COMPARING METRIC MEASUREMENTS

Example A

  i Change 0.4 L to mL.

  ii Change 0.04 L to mL.

 iii Which is larger: 0.4 L or 0.04 L?

1 L = 1000 mL

  i 0.4 L = 0.4 × 1000 mL = 400 mL

  ii 0.04 L = 0.04 × 1000 mL = 40 mL

 iii 0.4 L is larger than 0.04 L

Example B

  i Convert 4.3 kg to grams.

  ii Convert 4.03 kg to grams.

 iii Which is heavier: 4.3 kg or 4.03 kg?

1 kg = 1000 g

  i 4.3 kg = 4.3 × 1000 g = 4300 g

  ii 4.03 kg = 4.03 × 1000 g = 4030 g

 iii 4.3 kg is heavier than 4.03 kg

Exercise 1D *Change each given measurement to the smaller unit required. Then (c) choose the larger of the two given measurements.*

Change each measurement to millilitres (mL); choose the larger volume.

					Larger
1	**a**	0.1 L	**b**	0.01 L	**c**
2	**a**	0.003 L	**b**	0.3 L	**c**
3	**a**	0.05 L	**b**	0.005 L	**c**
4	**a**	0.047 L	**b**	0.47 L	**c**

Convert each measurement to milligrams (mg); choose the larger mass (or weight).

5	**a**	0.4 g	**b**	0.004 g	**c**
6	**a**	0.06 g	**b**	0.6 g	**c**
7	**a**	0.07 g	**b**	0.007 g	**c**
8	**a**	0.63 g	**b**	0.063 g	**c**

Rewrite each measurement in micrograms (mcg); choose the bigger mass (or weight).

9	**a**	0.002 mg	**b**	0.02 mg	**c**
10	**a**	0.9 mg	**b**	0.09 mg	**c**
11	**a**	0.001 mg	**b**	0.1 mg	**c**
12	**a**	0.58 mg	**b**	0.058 mg	**c**

Change each measurement to grams (g); choose the heavier mass (or weight).

13	**a**	1.5 kg	**b**	1.05 kg	**c**
14	**a**	2.08 kg	**b**	2.8 kg	**c**
15	**a**	0.95 kg	**b**	0.095 kg	**c**
16	**a**	3.35 kg	**b**	3.5 kg	**c**

MULTIPLICATION OF DECIMALS

Note
d.p. is used in the examples to stand for *decimal place(s)*.

Example A *Multiply*

a 8×4
b 0.8×4
c 0.8×0.4
d 0.08×0.04

a $8 \times 4 = 32$
b $0.8 \times 4 = 3.2$
1 d.p. + 0 d.p. $\Rightarrow$ 1 d.p.

c $0.8 \times 0.4 = 0.32$
1 d.p. + 1 d.p. $\Rightarrow$ 2 d.p.

d $0.08 \times 0.04 = 0.0032$
2 d.p. + 2 d.p. $\Rightarrow$ 4 d.p.

Example B *Multiply*

a 67×4
b 6.7×0.4
c 0.67×4
d 6.7×0.04

a $67 \times 4 = 268$
b $6.7 \times 0.4 = 2.68$
1 d.p. + 1 d.p. $\Rightarrow$ 2 d.p.

c $0.67 \times 4 = 2.68$
2 d.p. + 0 d.p. $\Rightarrow$ 2 d.p.

d $6.7 \times 0.04 = 0.268$
1 d.p. + 2 d.p. $\Rightarrow$ 3 d.p.

Example C *Multiply*

a 16×12
b 1.6×1.2
c 0.16×0.12
d 0.016×1.2

a $16 \times 12 = 192$
b $1.6 \times 1.2 = 1.92$
c $0.16 \times 0.12 = 0.0192$
d $0.016 \times 1.2 = 0.0192$

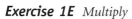

Exercise 1E *Multiply*

1 9×5
0.9×5
0.9×0.5
9×0.05

2 2×7
0.2×0.7
0.2×0.07
0.02×0.07

3 3×4
3×0.04
0.3×0.4
0.03×0.04

4 6×6
0.6×0.6
0.06×0.06
0.6×0.006

5 7×8
0.7×8
0.7×0.8
0.07×0.08

6 17×6
1.7×6
0.17×6
0.17×0.6

7 19×8
19×0.8
0.19×0.8
1.9×0.08

8 23×2
2.3×0.2
2.3×0.02
2.3×0.002

9 29×5
0.29×5
2.9×0.5
29×0.05

10 31×3
3.1×0.3
0.31×0.03
31×0.003

11 37×9
3.7×9
3.7×0.09
0.37×0.09

12 41×7
0.41×0.7
0.41×0.07
4.1×0.7

13 48×4
0.48×0.04
48×0.004
0.048×0.4

14 56×11
5.6×1.1
0.56×0.11
56×0.011

15 64×12
6.4×0.12
0.64×0.12
0.064×1.2

Check your answers on p 121

FACTORS

Many calculations involve the simplifying (or 'cancelling down') of fractions.

This requires a knowledge of *factors*. When a number is divided by one of its factors, the answer is a whole number (i.e. there is no remainder).

Example *Which of the numbers 2, 3, 5, 7, 11 are factors of 154?*

$$
\begin{array}{r} 77 \\ 2\overline{)154} \end{array}
\qquad
\begin{array}{r} 51\frac{1}{3} \\ 3\overline{)154} \end{array}
\qquad
\begin{array}{r} 30\frac{4}{5} \\ 5\overline{)154} \end{array}
\qquad
\begin{array}{r} 22 \\ 7\overline{)154} \end{array}
\qquad
\begin{array}{r} 14 \\ 11\overline{)154} \end{array}
$$

∴ 2, 7 and 11 are factors of 154.

Notes
- These are not the ONLY factors of 154.
- The numbers can, of course, be checked mentally!

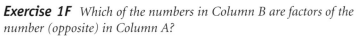

Exercise 1F *Which of the numbers in Column B are factors of the number (opposite) in Column A?*

	A	B
1	20	2, 3, 4, 5, 7, 8
2	36	3, 4, 5, 10, 12, 16
3	45	3, 5, 7, 11, 12, 15
4	56	2, 5, 8, 11, 14, 16
5	60	3, 4, 8, 12, 15, 20
6	72	3, 4, 6, 12, 15, 18
7	75	3, 5, 7, 11, 15, 25
8	85	3, 5, 9, 11, 15, 17
9	96	3, 8, 12, 14, 16, 24
10	100	3, 5, 8, 20, 25, 40
11	108	4, 7, 9, 12, 16, 18
12	120	3, 5, 9, 12, 15, 16
13	135	3, 5, 7, 9, 11, 15
14	144	4, 8, 12, 16, 18, 24
15	150	4, 5, 9, 12, 15, 25
16	165	3, 5, 7, 9, 11, 15
17	175	3, 5, 7, 9, 11, 15
18	180	4, 8, 12, 15, 16, 25
19	192	4, 6, 8, 12, 15, 16
20	210	4, 6, 9, 12, 14, 15

Check your answers on p 121

SIMPLIFYING FRACTIONS I

To simplify (or 'cancel down') a fraction, divide the numerator *and* the denominator by the *same* number. This number is called a *common factor*.

Note
The **numerator** is the top number in a fraction;
the **denominator** is the bottom number in that fraction.

Example A Simplify $\dfrac{36}{48}$

$$\frac{36}{48} = \frac{3}{4} \qquad \left[\begin{array}{l}\text{after dividing numerator and} \\ \text{denominator by 12}\end{array}\right]$$

Or this may be done in two or more steps:

$$\frac{36}{48} = \frac{18}{24} \qquad \left[\begin{array}{l}\text{dividing numerator and} \\ \text{denominator by 2}\end{array}\right]$$

$$= \frac{9}{12} \qquad \left[\begin{array}{l}\text{again dividing numerator and} \\ \text{denominator by 2}\end{array}\right]$$

$$= \frac{3}{4} \qquad \left[\begin{array}{l}\text{dividing numerator and} \\ \text{denominator by 3}\end{array}\right]$$

Note
$2 \times 2 \times 3 = 12$

Example B Simplify $\dfrac{125}{225}$

$$\frac{125}{225} = \frac{25}{45} \qquad \left[\begin{array}{l}\text{dividing numerator and} \\ \text{denominator by 5}\end{array}\right]$$

$$= \frac{5}{9} \qquad \left[\begin{array}{l}\text{again dividing numerator and} \\ \text{denominator by 5}\end{array}\right]$$

Exercise 1G

Part i *Simplify ('cancel down')*

1 $\dfrac{8}{12}$	**6** $\dfrac{15}{21}$	**11** $\dfrac{28}{32}$	**16** $\dfrac{14}{42}$	**21** $\dfrac{36}{56}$
2 $\dfrac{10}{14}$	**7** $\dfrac{20}{24}$	**12** $\dfrac{22}{33}$	**17** $\dfrac{30}{45}$	**22** $\dfrac{48}{60}$
3 $\dfrac{6}{16}$	**8** $\dfrac{20}{25}$	**13** $\dfrac{15}{35}$	**18** $\dfrac{42}{48}$	**23** $\dfrac{52}{64}$
4 $\dfrac{9}{18}$	**9** $\dfrac{12}{28}$	**14** $\dfrac{32}{36}$	**19** $\dfrac{36}{50}$	**24** $\dfrac{21}{70}$
5 $\dfrac{15}{20}$	**10** $\dfrac{9}{30}$	**15** $\dfrac{16}{40}$	**20** $\dfrac{25}{55}$	**25** $\dfrac{32}{72}$

Part ii *Simplify ('cancel down')*

1 $\dfrac{75}{150}$	**5** $\dfrac{125}{250}$	**9** $\dfrac{30}{225}$	**13** $\dfrac{125}{200}$	**17** $\dfrac{175}{225}$
2 $\dfrac{75}{200}$	**6** $\dfrac{125}{300}$	**10** $\dfrac{40}{175}$	**14** $\dfrac{375}{500}$	**18** $\dfrac{225}{300}$
3 $\dfrac{75}{250}$	**7** $\dfrac{125}{400}$	**11** $\dfrac{45}{150}$	**15** $\dfrac{275}{400}$	**19** $\dfrac{425}{600}$
4 $\dfrac{75}{300}$	**8** $\dfrac{125}{500}$	**12** $\dfrac{60}{375}$	**16** $\dfrac{100}{225}$	**20** $\dfrac{325}{750}$

SIMPLIFYING FRACTIONS II

Example A

Simplify $\dfrac{900}{1500}$

$\dfrac{900}{1500} = \dfrac{9}{15}$ $\left[\begin{array}{l}\text{dividing numerator and} \\ \text{denominator by 100}\end{array}\right]$

$\quad\ = \dfrac{3}{5}$ $\left[\begin{array}{l}\text{dividing numerator and} \\ \text{denominator by 3}\end{array}\right]$

Example B

Simplify $\dfrac{1400}{4000}$

$\dfrac{1400}{4000} = \dfrac{14}{40}$ $\left[\begin{array}{l}\text{dividing numerator and} \\ \text{denominator by 100}\end{array}\right]$

$\quad\ = \dfrac{7}{20}$ $\left[\begin{array}{l}\text{dividing numerator and} \\ \text{denominator by 2}\end{array}\right]$

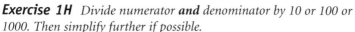

Exercise 1H *Divide numerator **and** denominator by 10 or 100 or 1000. Then simplify further if possible.*

1	$\dfrac{30}{50}$	**10**	$\dfrac{120}{160}$	**19**	$\dfrac{400}{600}$	**28**	$\dfrac{1400}{2500}$
2	$\dfrac{40}{60}$	**11**	$\dfrac{100}{160}$	**20**	$\dfrac{450}{600}$	**29**	$\dfrac{2000}{2500}$
3	$\dfrac{60}{80}$	**12**	$\dfrac{60}{160}$	**21**	$\dfrac{540}{600}$	**30**	$\dfrac{1750}{2500}$
4	$\dfrac{50}{120}$	**13**	$\dfrac{200}{300}$	**22**	$\dfrac{600}{800}$	**31**	$\dfrac{2500}{3000}$
5	$\dfrac{80}{120}$	**14**	$\dfrac{120}{300}$	**23**	$\dfrac{750}{800}$	**32**	$\dfrac{500}{3000}$
6	$\dfrac{100}{120}$	**15**	$\dfrac{270}{300}$	**24**	$\dfrac{320}{800}$	**33**	$\dfrac{450}{3000}$
7	$\dfrac{130}{150}$	**16**	$\dfrac{300}{500}$	**25**	$\dfrac{1000}{1500}$	**34**	$\dfrac{1500}{4000}$
8	$\dfrac{100}{150}$	**17**	$\dfrac{450}{500}$	**26**	$\dfrac{800}{1500}$	**35**	$\dfrac{1200}{4000}$
9	$\dfrac{60}{150}$	**18**	$\dfrac{120}{500}$	**27**	$\dfrac{1250}{1500}$	**36**	$\dfrac{2750}{4000}$

Check your answers on p 122

SIMPLIFYING FRACTIONS III

Leave answers as *improper fractions*.

Example A

Simplify $\dfrac{175}{50}$

$\dfrac{175}{50} = \dfrac{35}{10}$ $\quad\left[\begin{array}{l}\text{dividing numerator and} \\ \text{denominator by 5}\end{array}\right]$

$\phantom{\dfrac{175}{50}} = \dfrac{7}{2}$ $\quad\left[\begin{array}{l}\text{again dividing numerator and} \\ \text{denominator by 5}\end{array}\right]$

Example B

Simplify $\dfrac{400}{120}$

$\dfrac{400}{120} = \dfrac{40}{12}$ $\quad\left[\begin{array}{l}\text{dividing numerator and} \\ \text{denominator by 10}\end{array}\right]$

$\phantom{\dfrac{400}{120}} = \dfrac{10}{3}$ $\quad\left[\begin{array}{l}\text{dividing numerator and} \\ \text{denominator by 4}\end{array}\right]$

Exercise 1I *Simplify ('cancel down'). Leave answers as improper fractions.*

1 a $\dfrac{30}{20}$ b $\dfrac{50}{20}$ c $\dfrac{75}{20}$ d $\dfrac{85}{20}$

2 a $\dfrac{100}{8}$ b $\dfrac{150}{8}$ c $\dfrac{300}{8}$ d $\dfrac{750}{8}$

3 a $\dfrac{150}{12}$ b $\dfrac{350}{12}$ c $\dfrac{500}{12}$ d $\dfrac{1000}{12}$

4 a $\dfrac{100}{40}$ b $\dfrac{300}{40}$ c $\dfrac{380}{40}$ d $\dfrac{550}{40}$

5 a $\dfrac{70}{50}$ b $\dfrac{75}{50}$ c $\dfrac{120}{50}$ d $\dfrac{125}{50}$

6 a $\dfrac{80}{60}$ b $\dfrac{150}{60}$ c $\dfrac{750}{60}$ d $\dfrac{1000}{60}$

7 a $\dfrac{100}{80}$ b $\dfrac{200}{80}$ c $\dfrac{550}{80}$ d $\dfrac{1000}{80}$

8 a $\dfrac{180}{120}$ b $\dfrac{200}{120}$ c $\dfrac{300}{120}$ d $\dfrac{450}{120}$

9 a $\dfrac{200}{125}$ b $\dfrac{300}{125}$ c $\dfrac{800}{125}$ d $\dfrac{900}{125}$

10 a $\dfrac{150}{125}$ b $\dfrac{350}{125}$ c $\dfrac{550}{125}$ d $\dfrac{950}{125}$

11 a $\dfrac{180}{150}$ b $\dfrac{225}{150}$ c $\dfrac{400}{150}$ d $\dfrac{950}{150}$

12 a $\dfrac{800}{250}$ b $\dfrac{900}{250}$ c $\dfrac{1200}{250}$ d $\dfrac{1800}{250}$

SIMPLIFYING FRACTIONS IV

To simplify a fraction involving decimals, multiply the fraction by $\frac{10}{10}$ or $\frac{100}{100}$, depending on whether the *higher* (or *equal*) number of decimal places is 1 d.p. (then multiply by $\frac{10}{10}$) or 2 d.p. (then multiply by $\frac{100}{100}$). d.p. stands for *decimal place(s)*.

Example A   Simplify $\dfrac{0.4}{0.6}$ $\begin{array}{l} 0.4 \leftarrow 1 \text{ d.p.} \\ 0.6 \leftarrow 1 \text{ d.p.} \end{array}$ $\left[\begin{array}{l} \text{both numerator and} \\ \text{denominator have 1 d.p.} \end{array}\right]$

$$\frac{0.4}{0.6} \times \frac{10}{10} = \frac{4}{6} = \frac{2}{3}$$

Example B   Simplify $\dfrac{0.35}{0.4}$ $\begin{array}{l} 0.35 \leftarrow 2 \text{ d.p.} \\ 0.4 \leftarrow 1 \text{ d.p.} \end{array}$ $\left[\begin{array}{l} \text{numerator has 2 d.p.;} \\ \text{denominator has 1 d.p.} \end{array}\right]$

$$\frac{0.35}{0.4} \times \frac{100}{100} = \frac{35}{40} = \frac{7}{8}$$

Example C   Simplify $\dfrac{100}{2.5}$ $\begin{array}{l} 100 \leftarrow 0 \text{ d.p.} \\ 2.5 \leftarrow 1 \text{ d.p.} \end{array}$ $\left[\begin{array}{l} \text{numerator has 0 d.p.;} \\ \text{denominator has 1 d.p.} \end{array}\right]$

$$\frac{100}{2.5} \times \frac{10}{10} = \frac{1000}{25} = \frac{200}{5} = \frac{40}{1} = 40$$

Example D   Simplify $\dfrac{0.07}{0.02}$ $\begin{array}{l} 0.07 \leftarrow 2 \text{ d.p.} \\ 0.02 \leftarrow 2 \text{ d.p.} \end{array}$ $\left[\begin{array}{l} \text{both numerator and} \\ \text{denominator have 2 d.p.} \end{array}\right]$

$$\frac{0.07}{0.02} \times \frac{100}{100} = \frac{7}{2} \quad \left[\begin{array}{l} \text{leave answer as} \\ \text{an improper fraction} \end{array}\right]$$

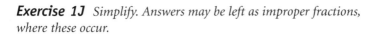

Exercise 1J *Simplify. Answers may be left as improper fractions, where these occur.*

Part i

1 $\dfrac{0.4}{0.5}$ 6 $\dfrac{0.35}{0.5}$ 11 $\dfrac{200}{2.5}$ 16 $\dfrac{0.09}{0.02}$

2 $\dfrac{0.6}{0.8}$ 7 $\dfrac{0.45}{0.2}$ 12 $\dfrac{100}{1.5}$ 17 $\dfrac{0.05}{0.04}$

3 $\dfrac{0.9}{0.6}$ 8 $\dfrac{0.55}{0.1}$ 13 $\dfrac{300}{1.5}$ 18 $\dfrac{0.04}{0.06}$

4 $\dfrac{0.3}{0.7}$ 9 $\dfrac{0.75}{0.3}$ 14 $\dfrac{100}{4.5}$ 19 $\dfrac{0.07}{0.01}$

5 $\dfrac{0.8}{0.4}$ 10 $\dfrac{0.95}{0.4}$ 15 $\dfrac{500}{5.5}$ 20 $\dfrac{0.04}{0.08}$

Part ii

1 $\dfrac{0.6}{0.4}$ 4 $\dfrac{200}{1.5}$ 7 $\dfrac{0.9}{0.1}$ 10 $\dfrac{0.05}{0.02}$

2 $\dfrac{0.03}{0.09}$ 5 $\dfrac{0.3}{0.6}$ 8 $\dfrac{300}{2.5}$ 11 $\dfrac{0.75}{0.5}$

3 $\dfrac{0.15}{0.2}$ 6 $\dfrac{0.06}{0.08}$ 9 $\dfrac{0.25}{0.4}$ 12 $\dfrac{100}{3.5}$

ROUNDING-OFF DECIMAL NUMBERS

Rounding-off to *one* decimal place

Method If the *second* decimal place is *5 or more* then *add one* to the first decimal place. If the second decimal place is *less than 5* then leave the first decimal place as it is.

Example A

Write   i 0.62   ii 1.75   iii 3.49 correct to one decimal place

i 0.6② ≈ 0.6   **ii** 1.7⑤ ≈ 1.8   **iii** 3.4⑨ ≈ 3.5

[The symbol ≈ stands for *is approximately equal to.*]

Rounding-off to *two* decimal places

Method If the *third* decimal place is *5 or more* then *add one* to the second decimal place. If the third decimal place is *less than 5* then leave the second decimal place as it is.

Example B

Write   i 0.827   ii 0.694   iii 2.145 correct to two decimal places

i 0.82⑦ ≈ 0.83   **ii** 0.69④ ≈ 0.69   **iii** 2.14⑤ ≈ 2.15

Rounding-off to *three* decimal places

Method If the *fourth* decimal place is *5 or more* then *add one* to the third decimal place. If the fourth decimal place is *less than 5* then leave the third decimal place as it is.

Example C

Write   i 0.7854   ii 1.5968   iii 0.9705 correct to three decimal places

i 0.785④ ≈ 0.785   **ii** 1.596⑧ ≈ 1.597   **iii** 0.970⑤ ≈ 0.971

Exercise 1K

Part i *Write each number correct to ONE decimal place.*

1 0.93	**5** 0.58	**9** 2.37	**13** 1.06
2 0.47	**6** 0.96	**10** 1.09	**14** 2.98
3 0.85	**7** 1.57	**11** 0.16	**15** 1.02
4 0.69	**8** 1.22	**12** 2.65	**16** 0.75

Part ii *Write each number correct to TWO decimal places.*

1 0.333	**5** 0.142	**9** 2.714	**13** 0.625
2 1.667	**6** 0.125	**10** 1.285	**14** 0.777
3 0.875	**7** 0.916	**11** 0.636	**15** 2.428
4 0.833	**8** 1.571	**12** 0.222	**16** 1.857

Part iii *Write each number correct to THREE decimal places.*

1 0.4863	**5** 1.5288	**9** 0.8155	**13** 3.0909
2 0.9547	**6** 0.3113	**10** 1.1196	**14** 0.1645
3 0.6060	**7** 2.8585	**11** 0.1652	**15** 2.7801
4 1.4145	**8** 0.1699	**12** 2.9625	**16** 1.7575

FRACTION TO A DECIMAL I

Some fractions have *exact* decimal equivalents; other fractions have only *approximate* decimal equivalents. The fractions in this exercise have *exact* decimal equivalents.

Example A

Change $\frac{2}{5}$ to a decimal.

Method   Divide the numerator by the denominator.

$5{\overline{)\,2.0}}$ ← *Write as many zeros as you need.*
$\quad 0.4$

$\therefore \frac{2}{5} = 0.4$

Example B

Change $\frac{3}{8}$ to a decimal.

$8{\overline{)\,3.0^60^40}}$ ← *Write as many zeros as you need.*
$\quad\ 0.375$

Example C

Change $\frac{3}{20}$ to a decimal.

$10{\overline{)\,3}}$
$\ 2{\overline{)\,0.3^10}}$ $\left[\begin{array}{l}\text{divide by 10}\\ \text{and then 2}\\ \text{since } 10 \times 2\ = 20\end{array}\right]$ *or* $\frac{3}{20} = \frac{15}{100}$
$\quad\ 0.15$ $\qquad\qquad\qquad\qquad\qquad\qquad = 0.15$

Example D

Change $\frac{14}{25}$ to a decimal.

$5{\overline{)\,14.^40}}$
$\ 2{\overline{)\ \,2.8^30}}$ $\left[\begin{array}{l}\text{divide by 5}\\ \text{and then 5 again}\\ \text{since } 5 \times 5\ = 25\end{array}\right]$ *or* $\frac{14}{25} = \frac{56}{100}$
$\quad\ 0.56$ $\qquad\qquad\qquad\qquad\qquad\qquad = 0.56$

Exercise 1L *Change each fraction to a decimal. All of these fractions have exact decimal equivalents. Refer to examples A and B.*

1 $\frac{1}{2}$	**3** $\frac{3}{4}$	**5** $\frac{3}{5}$	**7** $\frac{1}{8}$
2 $\frac{1}{4}$	**4** $\frac{1}{5}$	**6** $\frac{4}{5}$	**8** $\frac{7}{8}$

Change each fraction to a decimal. All of these fractions have exact decimal equivalents. Refer to examples C and D.

9 $\frac{1}{20}$	**13** $\frac{1}{25}$	**17** $\frac{1}{40}$	**21** $\frac{1}{50}$
10 $\frac{7}{20}$	**14** $\frac{8}{25}$	**18** $\frac{9}{40}$	**22** $\frac{7}{50}$
11 $\frac{13}{20}$	**15** $\frac{17}{25}$	**19** $\frac{11}{40}$	**23** $\frac{21}{50}$
12 $\frac{19}{20}$	**16** $\frac{22}{25}$	**20** $\frac{27}{40}$	**24** $\frac{43}{50}$

Check your answers on p 125

FRACTION TO A DECIMAL II

The fractions in this exercise have only *approximate* decimal equivalents.

Example A

Change $\frac{4}{7}$ to a decimal correct to ONE decimal place.

$$7)\ \overline{4.0^50}\quad \leftarrow \text{Use 2 zeros.}$$
$$\underline{\ 0.5\,⑦}$$

$$\therefore \frac{4}{7} \approx 0.6$$

[The symbol $\approx$ stands for *is approximately equal to*.]

Example B

Change $\frac{5}{6}$ to a decimal correct to TWO decimal places.

$$6)\ \overline{5.0^20^20}\quad \leftarrow \text{Use 3 zeros.}$$
$$\underline{\ 0.83\,③}$$

$$\therefore \frac{5}{6} \approx 0.83$$

Example C

Change $\frac{13}{60}$ to a decimal correct to THREE decimal places.

$$10)\ \overline{13.0}$$
$$6)\ \overline{1.3^10^40^40}\qquad \begin{bmatrix} \text{divide by 10} \\ \text{and then 6} \\ \text{since } 10 \times 6 = 60 \end{bmatrix}$$
$$\underline{\ 0.216\,⑥}$$

$$\therefore \frac{13}{60} \approx 0.217$$

Exercise 1M

Part i *Change each fraction to a decimal correct to ONE decimal place.*

1 $\dfrac{1}{3}$ **3** $\dfrac{2}{7}$ **5** $\dfrac{2}{9}$ **7** $\dfrac{6}{11}$

2 $\dfrac{5}{6}$ **4** $\dfrac{5}{7}$ **6** $\dfrac{3}{11}$ **8** $\dfrac{11}{12}$

Part ii *Change each fraction to a decimal correct to TWO decimal places.*

1 $\dfrac{2}{3}$ **3** $\dfrac{6}{7}$ **5** $\dfrac{8}{9}$ **7** $\dfrac{10}{11}$

2 $\dfrac{1}{6}$ **4** $\dfrac{4}{9}$ **6** $\dfrac{4}{11}$ **8** $\dfrac{5}{12}$

Part iii *Change each fraction to a decimal correct to THREE decimal places.*

1 $\dfrac{1}{30}$ **3** $\dfrac{7}{60}$ **5** $\dfrac{9}{70}$ **7** $\dfrac{1}{90}$

2 $\dfrac{17}{30}$ **4** $\dfrac{31}{60}$ **6** $\dfrac{53}{70}$ **8** $\dfrac{23}{90}$

FRACTION TO A DECIMAL III

Note
d.p. stands for *decimal place*.

Example A

Calculate the value of $\dfrac{175}{6}$ to the nearest whole number.

$$\frac{175}{6} = 175 \div 6$$

$$6 \overline{)17\,{}^{5}5.\,{}^{1}0} \atop 29.\,①$$

$$\therefore \frac{175}{6} \approx 29.1 \Rightarrow 29$$

If the first d.p. is 5 or more then add 1 to the whole number.

If the first d.p. is less than 5 then leave the whole number as it is.

Example B

Calculate the value of $\dfrac{7}{6}$ correct to one decimal place.

$$\frac{7}{6} = 7 \div 6$$

$$6 \overline{)7.\,{}^{1}0\,{}^{4}0} \atop 1.1\,⑥$$

$$\therefore \frac{7}{6} \approx 1.16 \Rightarrow 1.2$$

If the second d.p. is 5 or more then add 1 to the first d.p.

If the second d.p. is less than 5 then leave the first d.p. as it is.

Exercise 1N

Part i *Calculate the value of each fraction to the nearest whole number. Refer to example A.*

1 $\dfrac{100}{3}$ **5** $\dfrac{75}{4}$ **9** $\dfrac{125}{6}$ **13** $\dfrac{375}{8}$

2 $\dfrac{250}{3}$ **6** $\dfrac{125}{4}$ **10** $\dfrac{275}{6}$ **14** $\dfrac{425}{8}$

3 $\dfrac{500}{3}$ **7** $\dfrac{72}{5}$ **11** $\dfrac{240}{7}$ **15** $\dfrac{250}{9}$

4 $\dfrac{550}{3}$ **8** $\dfrac{144}{5}$ **12** $\dfrac{300}{7}$ **16** $\dfrac{550}{9}$

Part ii *Calculate the value of each fraction correct to one decimal place. Refer to example B.*

1 $\dfrac{5}{3}$ **5** $\dfrac{20}{7}$ **9** $\dfrac{25}{8}$ **13** $\dfrac{20}{9}$

2 $\dfrac{10}{3}$ **6** $\dfrac{25}{7}$ **10** $\dfrac{35}{8}$ **14** $\dfrac{50}{9}$

3 $\dfrac{35}{6}$ **7** $\dfrac{50}{7}$ **11** $\dfrac{55}{8}$ **15** $\dfrac{70}{9}$

4 $\dfrac{25}{6}$ **8** $\dfrac{65}{7}$ **12** $\dfrac{45}{8}$ **16** $\dfrac{85}{9}$

Check your answers on p 125

MIXED NUMBERS AND IMPROPER FRACTIONS

Example A

i Change $\dfrac{17}{5}$ to a mixed number.

$$\dfrac{17}{5} = 17 \div 5$$

$$= 3\tfrac{2}{5} \quad \leftarrow \text{remainder}$$
$$\quad\quad \leftarrow \text{same denominator as improper fraction}$$

ii Change $\dfrac{115}{4}$ to a mixed number.

$$\dfrac{115}{4} = 115 \div 4$$

$$= 28\tfrac{3}{4} \quad \leftarrow \text{remainder}$$
$$\quad\quad \leftarrow \text{same denominator as improper fraction}$$

Example B

i Change $8\tfrac{1}{4}$ to an improper fraction.

$$8\tfrac{1}{4} = \dfrac{33}{4} \quad \leftarrow 8 \times 4 + 1 = 33$$
$$\quad\quad\quad \leftarrow \text{same denominator as fraction in mixed number}$$

ii Change $20\tfrac{4}{5}$ to an improper fraction.

$$20\tfrac{4}{5} = \dfrac{104}{5} \quad \leftarrow 20 \times 5 + 4 = 104$$
$$\quad\quad\quad \leftarrow \text{same denominator as fraction in mixed number}$$

Exercise 10

Part i *Change these improper fractions to mixed numbers.*

1 $\frac{5}{2}$	**5** $\frac{29}{6}$	**9** $\frac{51}{2}$	**13** $\frac{95}{6}$	**17** $\frac{133}{5}$
2 $\frac{11}{3}$	**6** $\frac{36}{7}$	**10** $\frac{65}{3}$	**14** $\frac{101}{7}$	**18** $\frac{143}{6}$
3 $\frac{17}{4}$	**7** $\frac{37}{8}$	**11** $\frac{71}{4}$	**15** $\frac{113}{8}$	**19** $\frac{157}{7}$
4 $\frac{22}{5}$	**8** $\frac{49}{9}$	**12** $\frac{86}{5}$	**16** $\frac{125}{9}$	**20** $\frac{166}{9}$

Part ii *Rewrite these mixed numbers as improper fractions.*

1 $1\frac{1}{2}$	**5** $3\frac{1}{2}$	**9** $11\frac{1}{6}$	**13** $22\frac{1}{2}$	**17** $30\frac{5}{6}$
2 $1\frac{1}{3}$	**6** $4\frac{2}{3}$	**10** $13\frac{2}{7}$	**14** $24\frac{2}{3}$	**18** $32\frac{4}{7}$
3 $1\frac{3}{4}$	**7** $6\frac{1}{4}$	**11** $16\frac{5}{8}$	**15** $27\frac{3}{4}$	**19** $35\frac{3}{8}$
4 $2\frac{3}{5}$	**8** $9\frac{4}{5}$	**12** $17\frac{2}{9}$	**16** $29\frac{1}{5}$	**20** $38\frac{5}{9}$

MULTIPLICATION OF FRACTIONS

Example A $\dfrac{2}{5} \times \dfrac{4}{7}$

$$\dfrac{2}{5} \times \dfrac{4}{7} = \dfrac{2 \times 4}{5 \times 7}$$

$$= \dfrac{8}{35} \qquad \left[\begin{array}{l} \text{this fraction cannot} \\ \text{be simplified} \end{array} \right]$$

Example B $\dfrac{5}{8} \times \dfrac{7}{10}$

$$\dfrac{\overset{1}{\cancel{5}}}{8} \times \dfrac{7}{\underset{2}{\cancel{10}}} = \dfrac{1 \times 7}{8 \times 2} \qquad \left[\begin{array}{l} \text{note cancelling} \\ \text{across by 5} \end{array} \right]$$

$$= \dfrac{7}{16}$$

Example C $\dfrac{4}{9} \times \dfrac{21}{5}$

$$\dfrac{4}{\underset{3}{\cancel{9}}} \times \dfrac{\overset{7}{\cancel{21}}}{5} = \dfrac{4 \times 7}{3 \times 5} \qquad \left[\begin{array}{l} \text{note cancelling} \\ \text{across by 3} \end{array} \right]$$

$$= \dfrac{28}{15} \qquad \left[\begin{array}{l} \text{change this improper fraction} \\ \text{to a mixed number} \end{array} \right]$$

$$= 1\tfrac{13}{15} \qquad [\text{answer may be greater than one}]$$

Example D $\dfrac{9}{10} \times \dfrac{8}{15}$

$$\dfrac{\overset{3}{\cancel{9}}}{\underset{5}{\cancel{10}}} \times \dfrac{\overset{4}{\cancel{8}}}{\underset{5}{\cancel{15}}} = \dfrac{3 \times 4}{5 \times 5} \qquad \left[\begin{array}{l} \text{note cancelling across} \\ \text{by 3 and by 2} \end{array} \right]$$

$$= \dfrac{12}{25}$$

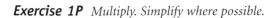

Exercise 1P *Multiply. Simplify where possible.*

1 $\frac{1}{2} \times \frac{2}{5}$

2 $\frac{1}{3} \times \frac{5}{8}$

3 $\frac{2}{3} \times \frac{5}{6}$

4 $\frac{1}{4} \times \frac{2}{3}$

5 $\frac{3}{4} \times \frac{20}{9}$

6 $\frac{1}{5} \times \frac{3}{10}$

7 $\frac{2}{5} \times \frac{3}{2}$

8 $\frac{3}{5} \times \frac{3}{4}$

9 $\frac{4}{5} \times \frac{25}{24}$

10 $\frac{1}{6} \times \frac{9}{10}$

11 $\frac{5}{6} \times \frac{8}{15}$

12 $\frac{1}{7} \times \frac{7}{18}$

13 $\frac{2}{7} \times \frac{11}{12}$

14 $\frac{3}{7} \times \frac{1}{20}$

15 $\frac{4}{7} \times \frac{5}{3}$

16 $\frac{5}{7} \times \frac{12}{25}$

17 $\frac{6}{7} \times \frac{5}{24}$

18 $\frac{1}{8} \times \frac{1}{2}$

19 $\frac{3}{8} \times \frac{12}{5}$

20 $\frac{5}{8} \times \frac{9}{20}$

21 $\frac{7}{8} \times \frac{8}{7}$

22 $\frac{1}{9} \times \frac{1}{15}$

23 $\frac{2}{9} \times \frac{7}{4}$

24 $\frac{4}{9} \times \frac{5}{12}$

25 $\frac{5}{9} \times \frac{21}{25}$

26 $\frac{7}{9} \times \frac{9}{16}$

27 $\frac{8}{9} \times \frac{1}{6}$

28 $\frac{1}{10} \times \frac{15}{8}$

29 $\frac{3}{10} \times \frac{4}{9}$

30 $\frac{7}{10} \times \frac{2}{7}$

31 $\frac{9}{10} \times \frac{15}{16}$

32 $\frac{1}{11} \times \frac{11}{18}$

33 $\frac{1}{12} \times \frac{1}{30}$

34 $\frac{5}{12} \times \frac{7}{30}$

35 $\frac{7}{12} \times \frac{9}{40}$

36 $\frac{11}{12} \times \frac{33}{40}$

Check your answers on p 126

2. Dosages of oral medications

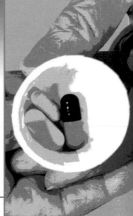

Drugs may be administered via several routes, including by injection, by intravenous infusion, or orally. The first medications that a student nurse will administer to patients are usually oral medications. Oral dosages may be in the form of tablets, capsules or liquid form.

A whole tablet is *always* preferable to a broken tablet because, unless a tablet is broken accurately, the dose will not be exact. If it is necessary to break a tablet or capsule, check the manufacturer's guidelines or check with the pharmacist to ensure it is acceptable to do so, as some should *never* be broken.

Many oral medications in liquid form are *suspensions*. These must be shaken thoroughly, in order to obtain the correct stock strength, before measuring out the required volume.

Check that stock strength and the strength required are given in the *same* unit in a particular calculation (i.e. *both* strengths in grams or milligrams or micrograms).

There are two symbols in use for microgram: μg and mcg. You may see both μg and mcg printed on drug charts. Doctors and nurses now more commonly use mcg, because if μg is written carelessly, then μg (for microgram) could be mistaken for mg (for milligram).

> **Important: If in *any* doubt about the answer to a calculation, then ask a supervisor to *check* your calculation.**

Example 1 *How many 50 mg tablets of atenolol should be given for a dose of atenolol 75 mg?*

$$\begin{aligned}\frac{\text{Volume}}{\text{required}} &= \frac{\text{Strength required}}{\text{Stock strength}} \times \left[\begin{array}{c}\text{Volume of}\\ \text{stock solution}\end{array}\right]\\ &= \frac{75 \text{ mg}}{50 \text{ mg}} \times 1 \text{ tablet}\\ &= \frac{3}{2} \text{ tablets}\\ &= 1\tfrac{1}{2} \text{ tablets}\end{aligned}$$

Note

In the case of tablets, "Volume required" refers to the number of tablets.

Example 2 *A patient is ordered 0.25 mg of digoxin, orally. The digoxin available is in tablets containing 125 mcg. How many such tablets should the patient receive?*

Change both strengths to the same units.

$$0.25 \text{ mg} = 250 \text{ mcg} \quad [\text{mcg} = \text{microgram}]$$

$$\begin{aligned}\therefore \frac{\text{Volume}}{\text{required}} &= \frac{\text{Strength required}}{\text{Stock strength}} \times \left[\begin{array}{c}\text{Volume of}\\ \text{stock solution}\end{array}\right]\\ &= \frac{250 \text{ mcg}}{125 \text{ mcg}} \times 1 \text{ tablet}\\ &= 2 \text{ tablets}\end{aligned}$$

Exercise 2A

1 A patient is ordered paracetamol 1 g, orally. Stock on hand is 500 mg tablets. Calculate the number of tablets required.

2 Ordered: codeine 15 mg, orally. Stock on hand: codeine tablets, 30 mg. How many tablets should the patient take?

3 A patient is ordered furosemide (frusemide) 60 mg, orally. In the ward are 40 mg tablets. How many tablets should be given?

4 How many 30 mg tablets of codeine are needed for a dose of 0.06 gram?

5 750 mg of ciprofloxacin is required. On hand are tablets of strength 500 mg. How many tablets should be given?

6 A patient is prescribed 150 mg of soluble aspirin. On hand are 300 mg tablets. What number should be given?

7 450 mg of soluble aspirin is ordered. Stock on hand is 300 mg tablets. How many tablets should the patient receive?

8 25 mg of captopril is prescribed. How many 50 mg tablets should be given?

9 The stock on hand of diazepam is 5 mg tablets. How many tablets are to be administered if the order is diazepam 12.5 mg?

10 Digoxin 125 mcg is ordered. Tablets available are 0.25 mg. How many tablets should be given?

---

*Check that you have used the **same unit of weight** throughout a calculation. Are **both** weights in milligrams (mg)?*
*Or are **both** weights in micrograms (mcg)?*

For some medications, tablets are available in different strengths. The tablets may be colour-coded to reduce the risk of error when dispensing.

Example 3 *Choose the best combination of 1 mg, 2 mg, 5 mg or 10 mg tablets of warfarin for each of these dosages:*

i 6 mg   ii 8 mg   iii 11 mg   iv 14 mg.

The number of tablets should be as few as possible and only whole tablets may be used.

   i 5 mg + 1 mg (2 tabs)

  ii 5 mg + 2 mg + 1 mg (3 tabs)

 iii 10 mg + 1 mg (2 tabs)

  iv 10 mg + 2 mg + 2 mg (3 tabs)

Exercise 2B *Choose the best combination of tablets for each of the following prescriptions. The **number** of tablets should be as few as possible and only **whole** tablets may be used.*

---

1 *Prescribed*: warfarin tablets
Strengths available: 1 mg, 2 mg, 5 mg, 10 mg
Dosages required: **a** 4 mg **b** 9 mg **c** 12 mg **d** 15 mg

2 *Prescribed*: diazepam tablets
Strengths available: 2 mg, 5 mg, 10 mg
Dosages required: **a** 7 mg **b** 9 mg **c** 15 mg **d** 20 mg

3 *Prescribed*: verapamil tablets
Strengths available: 40 mg, 80 mg, 120 mg, 160 mg
Dosages required: **a** 200 mg **b** 240 mg **c** 280 mg **d** 320 mg

4 *Prescribed*: prazosin tablets
Strengths available: 1 mg, 2 mg, 5 mg
Dosages required: **a** 6 mg **b** 8 mg **c** 9 mg **d** 11 mg

5 *Prescribed*: furosemide (frusemide) tablets
Strengths available: 20 mg, 40 mg, 80 mg, 500 mg
Dosages required: **a** 60 mg **b** 100 mg **c** 200 mg **d** 560 mg

6 *Prescribed*: thioridazine tablets
Strengths available: 10 mg, 25 mg, 50 mg, 100 mg
Dosages required: **a** 35 mg **b** 60 mg **c** 75 mg **d** 120 mg

---

Example 4 *A syrup contains penicillin 125 mg/5 mL. How many milligrams of penicillin are in   i 10 mL   ii 15 mL   iii 25 mL of the syrup?*

i 10 mL = 2 × 5 mL
   10 mL syrup contains 2 × 125 mg = 250 mg penicillin

ii 15 mL = 3 × 5 mL
   15 mL syrup contains 3 × 125 mg = 375 mg penicillin

iii 25 mL = 5 × 5 mL
   25 mL syrup contains 5 × 125 mg = 625 mg penicillin

Example 5 *A suspension contains paracetamol 120 mg/5 mL. How many milligrams of paracetamol are in   i 10 mL   ii 20 mL   iii 35 mL of the suspension?*

i 10mL = 2 × 5 mL
   10 mL suspension contains 2 × 120 mg = 240 mg paracetamol

ii 20 mL = 4 × 5 mL
   20 mL suspension contains 4 × 120 mg = 480 mg paracetamol

iii 35 mL = 7 × 5 mL
   35 mL suspension contains 7 × 120 mg = 840 mg paracetamol

Exercise 2C

1 A solution contains furosemide (frusemide) 10 mg/mL. How many milligrams of frusemide are in
    a 2 mL   **b** 3 mL   **c** 5 mL of the solution?

2 A solution contains morphine hydrochloride 2 mg/mL. How many milligrams of morphine hydrochloride are in
    a 3 mL   **b** 5 mL   **c** 7 mL of the solution?

3 Another solution contains morphine hydrochloride 40 mg/mL. How many milligrams of morphine hydrochloride are in
    a 2 mL   **b** 5 mL   **c** 10 mL of this solution?

4 A suspension contains phenytoin 125 mg/5 mL. How many milligrams of phenytoin are in
    a 20 mL   **b** 30 mL   **c** 40 mL of the suspension?

5 A solution contains fluoxetine 20 mg/5 mL. How many milligrams of fluoxetine are in
    a 10 mL   **b** 25 mL   **c** 40 mL of the solution?

6 A suspension contains erythromycin 250 mg/5 mL. How many milligrams of erythromycin are in
    a 10 mL   **b** 20 mL   **c** 30 mL of the suspension?

7 A syrup contains chlorpromazine 25 mg/5 mL. How many milligrams of chlorpromazine are in
    a 10 mL   **b** 30 mL   **c** 50 mL of the syrup?

8 A mixture contains penicillin 250 mg/5 mL. How many milligrams of penicillin are in
    a 15 mL   **b** 25 mL   **c** 35 mL of the mixture?

Example 6 *750 mg of erythromycin is to be given orally. Stock suspension contains 250 mg/5 mL. Calculate the volume to be given.*

$$\begin{aligned}
\frac{\text{Volume}}{\text{required}} &= \frac{\text{Strength required}}{\text{Stock strength}} \times \left[\begin{array}{c}\text{Volume of}\\\text{stock solution}\end{array}\right]\\[2mm]
&= \frac{750 \text{ mg}}{250 \text{ mg}} \times 5 \text{ mL}\\[2mm]
&= \frac{750}{250} \times \frac{5}{1}\text{mL}\\[2mm]
&= \frac{3}{1} \times \frac{5}{1}\text{mL} \left[\text{after simplifying } \frac{750}{250}\right]\\[2mm]
&= 15 \text{ mL}
\end{aligned}$$

Example 7 *A patient is ordered 800 mg of penicillin, orally. Stock on hand has a strength of 250 mg/5 mL. Calculate the volume required.*

$$\begin{aligned}
\frac{\text{Volume}}{\text{required}} &= \frac{\text{Strength required}}{\text{Stock strength}} \times \left[\begin{array}{c}\text{Volume of}\\\text{stock solution}\end{array}\right]\\[2mm]
&= \frac{800 \text{ mg}}{250 \text{ mg}} \times 5 \text{ mL}\\[2mm]
&= \frac{800}{250} \times \frac{5}{1}\text{mL}\\[2mm]
&= \frac{16}{5} \times \frac{5}{1}\text{mL} \left[\text{after simplifying } \frac{800}{250}\right]\\[2mm]
&= 16 \text{ mL}
\end{aligned}$$

Exercise 2D *In each example, you are given the prescribed dosage and the strength of stock on hand. Calculate the volume to be given.*

1 Ordered : penicillin 500 mg
   On hand : syrup 125 mg/5 mL

2 Ordered : furosemide (frusemide) 40 mg
   On hand : solution 10 mg/mL

3 Ordered : morphine hydrochloride 100 mg
   On hand : solution 40 mg/mL

4 Ordered : paracetamol 180 mg
   On hand : suspension 120 mg/5 mL

5 Ordered : phenytoin 150 mg
   On hand : suspension 125 mg/5 mL

6 Ordered : erythromycin 1250 mg
   On hand : suspension 250 mg/5 mL

7 Ordered : fluoxetine 30 mg
   On hand : solution 20 mg/5 mL

8 Ordered : penicillin 1000 mg
   On hand : mixture 250 mg/5 mL

9 Ordered : chlorpromazine 35 mg
   On hand : syrup 25 mg/5 mL

10 Ordered : penicillin 1200 mg
   On hand : mixture 250 mg/5 mL

11 Ordered : erythromycin 800 mg
   On hand : mixture 125 mg/5 mL

Exercise 2E *Read each label carefully.*

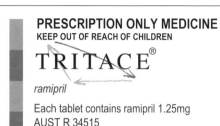

PRESCRIPTION ONLY MEDICINE
KEEP OUT OF REACH OF CHILDREN

TRITACE®

ramipril

Each tablet contains ramipril 1.25mg
AUST R 34515
30 Tablets

1.25mg

⁂*Aventis*

1 A patient is ordered ramipril 2.5 mg orally. How many of these
   Tritace tablets should be given?

PRESCRIPTION ONLY MEDICINE
KEEP OUT OF REACH OF CHILDREN

METRONIDE® 200

Metronidazole Tablets
21 TABLETS
Each tablet contains METRONIDAZOLE 200mg
AUST R 65540

2 How many Metronide 200 tablets should be given for an order
   of metronidazole 400 mg orally?

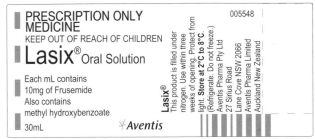

PRESCRIPTION ONLY MEDICINE

KEEP OUT OF REACH OF CHILDREN

Lasix® Oral Solution

Each mL contains
10mg of Frusemide
Also contains
methyl hydroxybenzoate

30mL

⚹ *Aventis*

005548

Lasix®
This product is filled under nitrogen. Use within three weeks of opening. Protect from light. **Store at 2°C to 8°C.** (Refrigerate. Do not freeze.) Aventis Pharma Pty Ltd
27 Sirius Road
Lane Cove NSW 2066
Aventis Pharma Limited
Auckland New Zealand

3   **a**   How many mg of furosemide (frusemide) in
    i   1 mL
    ii   2 mL of Lasix Oral Solution?
  b   Calculate the volume required for a dose of furosemide (frusemide) 40 mg.

PRESCRIPTION ONLY MEDICINE
KEEP OUT OF REACH OF CHILDREN

Largactil® Syrup

chlorpromazine hydrochloride

25mg

Chlorpromazine oral solution
Each 5mL contains 25mg
chlorpromazine hydrochloride

100mL syrup

⚹ *Aventis*

Largactil® Syrup
Contact with the skin should be avoided by those handling Largactil preparations to minimise the risk of dermatitis.

This medicine may cause drowsiness and may increase the effects of alcohol. If affected, do not drive or operate machinery.

DOSAGE: As directed by physician.
Store below 25°C. Protect from light.

Aventis Pharma Pty Ltd
27 Sirius Road
Lane Cove NSW 2066
Australia

005905

4   **a**   How many mg of chlorpromazine in
    i   5 mL
    ii   10 mL of Largactil Syrup?
  b   Calculate the volume required for a dose of chlorpromazine 40 mg.

CHAPTER 2 Revision

1 A patient is ordered penicillin 500 mg orally. In the ward are 250 mg capsules. What number should be given?

2 12.5 mg of captopril is prescribed for hypertension. On hand are tablets of strength 25 mg. How many tablets should be given?

3 How many 30 mg tablets of codeine should be given for a dose of codeine 45 mg?

4 Choose the best combination of 1 mg, 2 mg, 5 mg and 10 mg tablets of warfarin for each of these dosages:
  a 3 mg   **b** 7 mg   **c** 13 mg   **d** 16 mg

5 Many oral medications in liquid form are suspensions. What must be done to those medications before measuring out the required volume?

6 A solution contains furosemide (frusemide) 10 mg/mL. How many milligrams of frusemide are in
  a 5 mL   **b** 10 mL   **c** 25mL of the solution?

7 A suspension contains erythromycin 250mg/5mL. How many milligrams of erythromycin are in
  a 15 mL   **b** 25 mL   **c** 35 mL of the suspension?

8 A patient is ordered 750 mg of erythromycin, orally. Calculate the volume required if the suspension on hand has a strength of 250 mg/5 mL.

9 Paracetamol 750 mg is to be given as a syrup. Stock on hand contains 150 mg in 5 mL. Calculate the volume of syrup to be given.

10 A patient is prescribed penicillin 400 mg, orally. Stock syrup has a strength of 125 mg/5 mL. What volume should be given?

11 Flucloxacillin 375 mg is ordered. Stock syrup contains 125 mg/ 5 mL. What volume of syrup should the patient be given?

12 Furosemide (frusemide) 125 mg is ordered. Stock solution is 50 mg/mL. What volume of solution should be given?

3. Drug dosages for injection

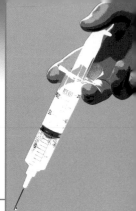

Correct measurement of drug dosages for injection is essential. An overdose can be dangerous; too low a dose may result in a drug being ineffective.

The number of decimal places in each answer should relate to the graduations on the syringe being used. Syringes with a capacity of more than 1 mL are usually graduated in tenths or fifths of a millilitre: so for volumes *greater* than 1 mL calculate answers to *one* decimal place. Syringes with a capacity of 1 mL or less are often graduated in hundredths of a millilitre: so for volumes *less* than 1 mL calculate answers to *two* decimal places.

Remember that there are *two* symbols in use for microgram: µg and mcg.

Also remember to check that stock strength *and* the strength required are given in the same units in a particular problem.

> *If in any doubt about the answer to a calculation, then ask a supervisor to check your calculation.*

Example 1 *Pethidine 75 mg is to be given I.M.I. Stock ampoules of pethidine contain 100 mg in 2 mL. Is the volume to be drawn up for injection equal to 2 mL, less than 2 mL, or more than 2 mL?*

A stock ampoule contains 100 mg of pethidine.
Volume of ampoule = 2 mL
75 mg (prescribed) is *less than* 100 mg (ampoule).
Therefore, volume to be drawn up is *less than* 2 mL.

Example 2 *Vancomycin 1200 mg is ordered. Stock vials contain vancomycin 1 g/10 mL (once diluted). Is the volume of stock required for injection equal to 10 mL, less than 10 mL, or more than 10 mL?*

A stock vial contains 1 g of vancomycin.
1 g = 1 gram = 1000 mg
Volume of vial = 10 mL
1200 mg (prescribed) is *more than* 1000 mg (vial).
Therefore, volume required is *more than* 10 mL.

Example 3 *A patient is to be given 12 000 units of Calciparine. Available ampoules contain 25 000 units in 1 mL. Should the volume to be drawn up for injection be equal to 1 mL, less than 1 mL, or more than 1 mL?*

A stock ampoule contains 25 000 units.
Volume of ampoule = 1 mL
12 000 units (prescribed) is *less than* 25 000 units (ampoule).
Therefore, volume to be drawn up is *less than* 1 mL.

Exercise 3A *Rewrite the correct answer to each problem. The answer will be either equal to, less than, or more than the volume of the stock ampoule or vial.*

1 An injection of morphine 9 mg is ordered. A stock ampoule contains morphine 15 mg in 1 mL. The volume to be drawn up for injection will be equal to 1 mL/less than 1 mL/more than 1 mL.

2 A patient is to receive an injection of ondansetron 6 mg. Stock ampoules contain ondansetron 4 mg/2 mL. The volume to be drawn up for injection is equal to 2 mL/less than 2 mL/more than 2 mL.

3 Furosemide (frusemide) 80 mg is ordered. Ampoules contain furosemide (frusemide) 250 mg in 5 mL. The volume required for injection is equal to 5 mL/less than 5 mL/more than 5 mL.

4 Benzylpenicillin 1.2 g is ordered. Stock vials contain 600 mg in 2 mL, when diluted. The volume of stock required is equal to 2 mL/less than 2 mL/more than 2 mL.

5 A patient is prescribed flucloxacillin 1000 mg, I.V. If stock ampoules contain 1 g in 10 mL, once diluted, then the amount of stock solution to be drawn up will be equal to 10 mL/less than 10 mL/more than 10 mL.

6 On hand are digoxin ampoules containing 500 mcg in 2 mL. An injection of 225 mcg is ordered. The volume required is equal to 2 mL/less than 2 mL/more than 2 mL.

7 Heparin is available at a strength of 1000 units per mL. The volume needed to give 1250 units is equal to 1 mL/less than 1 mL/more than 1 mL.

8 Diazepam 15 mg is to be given, I.V. Stock ampoules contain 10 mg in 2 mL. The volume to be drawn up is equal to 2 mL/less than 2 mL/more than 2 mL.

Think carefully about each answer in the exercises that follow. Should the volume to be drawn up for injection be equal to, less than, or more than the volume of the stock ampoule?

Example 4 *A patient is ordered furosemide (frusemide) 60 mg, I.V. Ampoules contain furosemide (frusemide) 80 mg in 2 mL. Calculate the volume required for injection.*

$$\begin{aligned}\text{Volume required} &= \frac{\text{Strength required}}{\text{Stock strength}} \times \left[\begin{array}{c}\text{Volume of}\\\text{stock solution}\end{array}\right]\\[2mm]
&= \frac{60\text{ mg}}{80\text{ mg}} \times 2\text{ mL}\\[2mm]
&= \frac{60}{80} \times \frac{2}{1}\text{ mL}\\[2mm]
&= \frac{3}{2}\text{ mL or 1.5 mL}\end{aligned}$$

Simplifying : $\dfrac{60}{80} \times \dfrac{2}{1} = \dfrac{3}{4} \times \dfrac{2}{1} = \dfrac{6}{4} = \dfrac{3}{2}$

Example 5 *An injection of digoxin 175 mcg is ordered. Stock on hand is digoxin 500 mcg in 2 mL. What volume of stock solution should be given?*

$$\begin{aligned}\text{Volume required} &= \frac{\text{Strength required}}{\text{Stock strength}} \times \left[\begin{array}{c}\text{Volume of}\\\text{stock solution}\end{array}\right]\\[2mm]
&= \frac{175\text{ mcg}}{500\text{ mcg}} \times 2\text{ mL}\\[2mm]
&= \frac{175}{500} \times \frac{2}{1}\text{ mL}\\[2mm]
&= \frac{7}{10}\text{ mL or 0.7 mL}\end{aligned}$$

Simplifying : $\dfrac{175}{500} \times \dfrac{2}{1} = \dfrac{7}{20} \times \dfrac{2}{1} = \dfrac{14}{20} = \dfrac{7}{10}$

Note
mcg = microgram
Stock strength refers to the strength of the medication supplied.

Exercise 3B

1 An injection of morphine 8 mg is required. Ampoules on hand contain 10 mg in 1 mL. What volume is drawn up for injection?

2 Digoxin ampoules on hand contain 500 mcg in 2 mL. What volume is needed to give 350 mcg?

3 A child is ordered 9 mg of gentamicin by I.M.I. Stock ampoules contain 20 mg in 2 mL. What volume is needed for the injection?

4 A patient is to be given flucloxacillin 250 mg by injection. Stock vials contain 1 g in 10 mL, after dilution. Calculate the required volume.

5 Stock heparin has a strength of 5000 units per mL. What volume must be drawn up to give 6500 units?

6 Pethidine 85 mg is to be given I.M. Stock ampoules contain pethidine 100 mg in 2 mL. Calculate the volume of stock required.

7 A patient is to receive an injection of gentamicin 60 mg, I.M. Ampoules on hand contain 80 mg/2 mL. Calculate the volume required.

8 A patient is prescribed naloxone 0.6 mg, I.V. Stock ampoules contain 0.4 mg/2 mL. What volume should be drawn up for injection?

Think about each answer. Does it make sense? Is it ridiculously large?

Exercise 3C

1 Vancomycin 500 mg is ordered. Stock on hand contains 1 g in 10 mL, once diluted. What volume is required?

2 A patient is to receive an I.V. dose of gentamicin 160 mg. Stock ampoules contain 100 mg in 2 mL. Calculate the volume to be drawn up for injection.

3 How much morphine solution must be withdrawn for a 7.5 mg dose if a stock ampoule contains 15 mg in 1 mL?

4 A patient is ordered 200 mg of furosemide (frusemide). Stock is 250 mg in 5 mL. Calculate the volume that is needed for injection.

5 Heparin is available at a strength of 5000 units/5 mL. What volume is needed to give 800 units?

6 Phenobarbitone 40 mg has been ordered. Stock ampoules contain 200 mg/mL. What volume should be given?

7 A patient is ordered pethidine 65 mg. Stock ampoules of pethidine contain 100 mg in 2 mL. Calculate the volume to be drawn up for injection.

8 A patient is to be given ranitidine 40 mg, I.V. Stock ampoules have a strength of 50 mg/2 mL. What volume of stock should be injected?

9 Morphine 5.5 mg is prescribed. Stock ampoules contain 10 mg/mL. What volume should be drawn up for injection?

Exercise 3D *Calculate the volume of stock to be drawn up for injection.*

---

1 Pethidine 60 mg is ordered. Stock ampoules contain 100 mg in 2 mL.

2 An adult is ordered metoclopramide 15 mg, for nausea. On hand are ampoules containing 10 mg/mL.

3 A patient is prescribed erythromycin 250 mg, I.V. Stock on hand contains 1 g in 10 mL, once diluted.

4 Tramadol hydrochloride 80 mg is required. Available stock contains 100 mg in 2 mL.

5 A patient is ordered benzylpenicillin 800 mg. On hand is benzylpenicillin 1.2 g in 6 mL.

6 An adult patient with TB is to be given 500 mg of capreomycin every second day, I.M.I. Stock on hand contains 1 g in 3 mL.

7 Digoxin ampoules on hand contain 500 mcg in 2 mL. Digoxin 150 mcg is ordered.

8 Stock Calciparine contains 25 000 units in 1 mL. 15 000 units of Calciparine are ordered.

9 Penicillin 450 mg is ordered. Stock ampoules contain 600 mg in 5 mL.

Exercise 3E *Calculate the amount of stock solution to be drawn up for injection. Give answers greater than 1 mL correct to one decimal place; answers less than 1 mL correct to two decimal places. If the next decimal place is 5 or more, add one to the previous digit.*

1 Ordered : erythromycin 200 mg
        Stock : 300 mg in 10 mL

2 Ordered : morphine 20 mg
        Stock : 15 mg in 1 mL

3 Ordered : atropine 0.5 mg
        Stock : 0.6 mg in 1 mL

4 Ordered : atropine 800 mcg
        Stock : 1.2 mg in 1 mL

5 Ordered : naloxone 0.35 mg
        Stock : 0.4 mg/mL

6 Ordered : capreomycin 850 mg
        Stock : 2 g per mL

7 Ordered : metoclopramide 7 mg
        Stock : 10 mg/2 mL

8 Ordered : heparin 1750 units
        Stock : 1000 units per mL

9 Ordered : buscopan 0.25 mg
        Stock : 0.4 mg/2 mL

Check your answers on p 129

Exercise 3F *Calculate the volume of stock required. Give answers greater than 1 mL correct to one decimal place; answers less than 1 mL correct to two decimal places.*

	Ordered		*Stock ampoule*
1	Morphine	12 mg	15 mg/mL
2	Calciparine	7000 units	25 000 units in 1 mL
3	Benzylpenicillin	1500 mg	1.2 g in 10 mL
4	Heparin	3000 units	5000 units/mL
5	Phenobarbitone	70 mg	200 mg/mL
6	Pethidine	80 mg	100 mg/2 mL
7	Buscopan	0.24 mg	0.4 mg/2 mL
8	Digoxin	200 mcg	500 mcg in 2 mL
9	Furosemide (frusemide)	150 mg	250 mg in 5 mL
10	Ondansetron	5 mg	4 mg in 2 mL
11	Capreomycin	800 mg	1 g in 5 mL
12	Tramadol	120 mg	100 mg in 2 mL
13	Gentamicin	70 mg	80 mg in 2 mL
14	Vancomycin	800 mg	1 g in 5 mL
15	Morphine	7.5 mg	10 mg in 1 mL
16	Ceftriaxone	1250 mg	1 g/3 mL
17	Buscopan	25 mg	20 mg in 1 mL
18	Dexamethasone	3 mg	4 mg/mL
19	Vancomycin	1.2 g	1000 mg/5 mL
20	Naloxone	0.5 mg	0.4 mg/mL

Exercise 3G Read each label carefully. Each label refers to the stock available on the ward.

1   A patient is to receive 8 mg of ondansetron I.V. Calculate what volume of Zofran should be drawn up.

PRESCRIPTION ONLY MEDICINE
KEEP OUT OF REACH OF CHILDREN

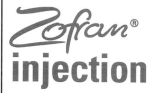

injection

ONDANSETRON
(AS HYDROCHLORIDE DIHYDRATE)
4 mg in 2 mL

5 x 2 mL Flexi-amp® ampoules

For slow intravenous administration.
In postoperative nausea and vomiting
the intramuscular route may be used.

AUST R 9978

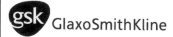 GlaxoSmithKline

www.gsk.com.au/zofran

2 Furosemide (frusemide) 60 mg I.V. has been prescribed for a patient. Calculate the volume of Lasix required.

PRESCRIPTION ONLY MEDICINE
KEEP OUT OF REACH OF CHILDREN

Lasix® **40**mg in **4**mL

frusemide injection

Diuretic
Solution for intravenous
or intramuscular injection

AUST R 76767

5 ampoules of **4** mL

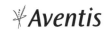

---

3 A patient has been ordered an injection of promethazine 12.5 mg I.M. What volume of Phenergan is required?

PRESCRIPTION ONLY MEDICINE
KEEP OUT OF THE REACH OF CHILDREN

PHENERGAN ®

Promethazine Injection
Promethazine Hydrochloride
25 mg in 1 mL
10 x 1 mL ampoules
For IM or IV Injection

AUST R 27545

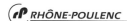
RHÔNE-POULENC

Rhône–Poulenc Rorer

4 35 mg of I.V. furosemide (frusemide) is ordered. How much Lasix should be drawn up for injection?

PRESCRIPTION ONLY MEDICINE
KEEP OUT OF REACH OF CHILDREN

Lasix®

frusemide injection

20mg in **2**mL

Diuretic
Solution for intravenous
or intramuscular injection
AUST R 12404
5 ampoules of **2** mL

Aventis

Exercise 3H *The drawings represent syringes (needles not shown).*

1 For this set of 1 mL syringes, write down the volume (mL) of solution
   a between adjacent graduations
   b indicated by arrows A, B, C and D.

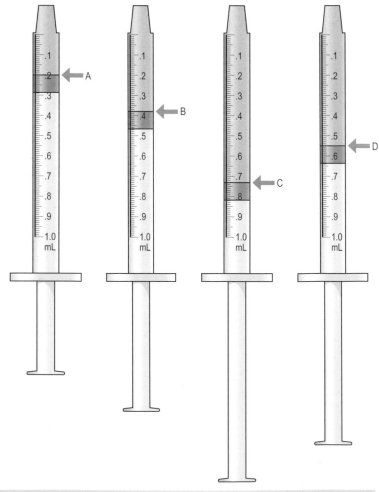

2 Note that these four syringes are graduated in **units**, especially for **insulin** injections. Write down the number of units of solution
  a between adjacent graduations
  b indicated by arrows A, B, C and D.

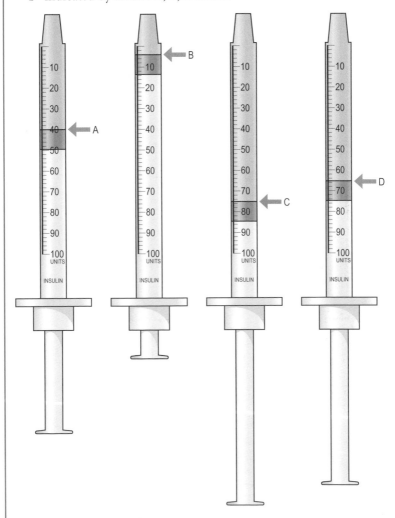

3 For this set of three syringes, write down the volume (mL) of solution
   a between adjacent graduations
   b indicated by arrows A, B and C.

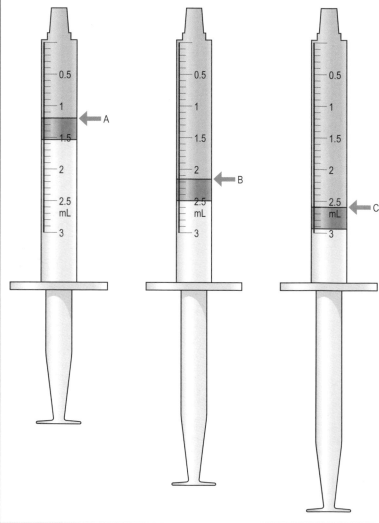

4 For these syringes, write down the volume (mL) of solution
   a between adjacent graduations
   b indicated by arrows A, B and C.

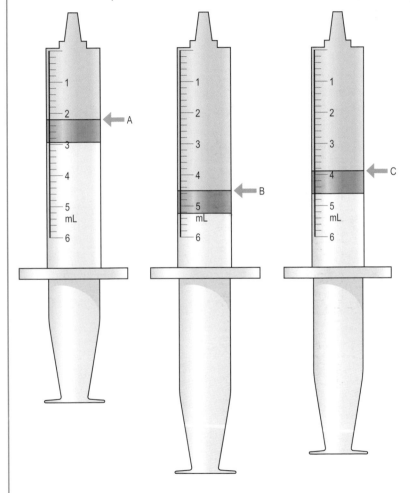

CHAPTER 3 Revision

1 Phenobarbitone 60 mg is to be given I.M.I. Stock ampoules contain 200 mg/mL. Is the volume of stock required equal to 1 mL, less than 1 mL, or more than 1 mL?

2 Pethidine 70 mg is to be given I.M.I. Calculate the volume of stock required if ampoules contain pethidine 100 mg in 2 mL.

3 Heparin 12 000 units, S.C., is ordered. Stock ampoules contain 25 000 units/5 mL. What volume should be drawn up?

4 A patient is ordered benzylpenicillin 900 mg. On hand is benzylpenicillin 600 mg in 5 mL (once diluted). Calculate the volume to be drawn up for injection.

5 Digoxin ampoules on hand contain 500 mcg in 2 mL. What volume is needed for an injection of 275 mcg?

6 A patient is ordered tramadol hydrochloride 75 mg, I.M.I. Ampoules contain tramadol hydrochloride 100 mg in 2 mL. Calculate the volume required for injection.

7 A patient is prescribed vancomycin 900 mg, I.V. Calculate the amount of stock solution required if stock on hand contains 1 g per 10 mL.

8 Buscopan 0.18 mg is ordered. Stock ampoules contain 0.4 mg/2 mL. Calculate the volume to be drawn up for injection.

9 A patient is to be given an injection of erythromycin 190 mg. Stock ampoules contain 300 mg/10 mL. Calculate the required volume.

10 How much morphine must be drawn up for a 10 mg dose if a stock ampoule contains 15 mg in 1 mL?

Check your answers on p 130

4. Intravenous infusion

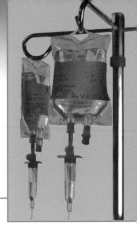

This chapter deals with the arithmetic of flow rates and drip rates for intravenous (I.V.) infusion.

The fluid being infused passes from a flask (or similar container) into a giving set (administration set) which has a drip chamber. The giving set may be free-hanging or attached to a volumetric infusion pump.

If the giving set is free-hanging, the nurse needs to calculate the drops per minute to be infused. The nurse can then manipulate the roller clamp on the giving set and ensure the drip rate is correct.

By contrast, if the giving set is connected to an infusion pump, then the nurse only needs to calculate the number of millilitres per hour to be infused and set the pump accordingly.

Note: There may be a burette between the flask and the giving set. The use of a burette will depend on institution policy and the type of infusion being used.

There are two main types of giving sets in general use – these break fluid into either 20 or 60 drops per mL. A drip chamber that delivers 60 drops per mL is also known as a *microdrip*.

Example 1 *A patient is receiving dextrose 5% by I.V. infusion. The drip rate is set to deliver 45 mL per hour. How much fluid will the patient receive over   i 2 h   ii 3h   iii 7 h?*

Volume (mL) = Rate (mL/h) × Time (h)

i 45mL/h × 2 h = 90 mL

ii 45 mL/h × 3 h = 135 mL

iii 45 mL/h × 7 h = 315 mL

Example 2 *A teenager is to receive 750 mL of Hartmann's solution. An infusion pump is set at 60 mL/h. How long will it take to give the solution?*

$$\text{Time (h)} = \frac{\text{Volume (mL)}}{\text{Rate (mL/h)}}$$

$$= \frac{750 \text{ mL}}{60 \text{ mL/h}}$$

$$= 12\tfrac{1}{2} \text{ hours or 12 h 30 min}$$

Simplifying : $\dfrac{750}{60} = \dfrac{75}{6} = \dfrac{25}{2} = 12\tfrac{1}{2}$

Exercise 4A

1 An intravenous line has been inserted in a patient. Fluid is being delivered at a rate of 42 mL/h. How much fluid will the patient receive in   **a** 2 h   **b** 8 h   **c** 12 h?

2 A male patient is receiving Hartmann's solution at a rate of 125 mL/h. How much solution will he receive over   **a** 3 h   **b** 5 h   **c** 12 h?

3 A girl is to be given dextrose 5% via an infusion pump. If the pump is set at 60 mL/h, how much dextrose 5% will she receive in   **a** $1\frac{1}{2}$ h   **b** $2\frac{1}{2}$ h   **c** 12 h?

4 A female patient is to receive 500 mL of normal saline. The drip rate is adjusted to deliver 25 mL/h. How long will the fluid last?

5 A young man is to be given one litre of dextrose 4% in $\frac{1}{5}$ normal saline. The infusion pump is set at a rate of 80 mL/h. What time will it take to give the litre of solution?

6 Half a litre of normal saline with 2 g potassium chloride is to be given to a patient I.V. How long will this take if the infusion pump is set at 75 mL/h?

7 A patient is to receive 100 mL of normal saline, I.V. If the infusion pump is set to deliver 150 mL/h, how long will the infusion take?

Example 3 *A patient is to receive half a litre of fluid I.V. over 6 hours using an infusion pump. At how many millilitres per hour should the pump be set? The pump does not have a decimal setting so calculate answer to the nearest whole number.*

Half a litre $= 500$ mL

Rate (mL/h) $= \dfrac{\text{Volume (mL)}}{\text{Time (h)}}$

$= \dfrac{500 \text{ mL}}{6 \text{ h}}$

$= \dfrac{250}{3} \text{mL/h}$

$\Rightarrow 83$ mL/h (to nearest whole number)

$$3 \overline{)25\,^{1}0.\,^{1}0}$$
$$\underline{83.\,\text{\textcircled{3}}}$$

Exercise 4B *Calculate the required flow rate of a volumetric infusion pump for each of the following infusions. Give answers in mL/h to the nearest whole number.*

1 One litre of normal saline is to be given over 8 hours.

2 A patient is to receive 500 mL of dextrose 5% over 12 hours.

3 500 mL of Hartmann's solution is to be given to a teenager over 7 hours.

4 Over the next 15 hours, a female patient is to receive 2 L of dextrose 4% in $\frac{1}{5}$ normal saline.

5 A teenager is to receive one litre of normal saline over 6 hours.

6 A woman is to be given 500 mL of dextrose 5% over 8 hours.

7 Over a period of 16 hours, a patient is to receive one litre of dextrose 4% in $\frac{1}{5}$ normal saline.

8 A patient is to be given one litre of normal saline over 24 hours.

9 80 mL of fluid in a burette is to be infused over half an hour.

10 A young man is to be given 100 mL of metronidazole 500 mg over half an hour.

Note: Half an hour = 0.5 h (if calculating flow rate using time in hours)
= 30 min (if calculating flow rate using time in minutes)
[See Exercise 4C]

Note: 60 minutes = 1 hour
60 min = 1 h

$$Rate\ (mL/min) = \frac{Volume\ (mL)}{Time\ (min)}$$

$$Rate\ (mL/h) = Rate\ (mL/min) \times 60$$

$$\therefore\ Rate\ (mL/h) = \frac{Volume\ (mL) \times 60}{Time\ (min)}$$

This method is used when infusion times are given in minutes.

Example 4 *75mL of fluid in a burette needs to be infused over 20 minutes. Calculate the flow rate required in mL/h. Give the answer to the nearest whole number.*

$$Rate\ (mL/h) = \frac{Volume\ (mL) \times 60}{Time\ (min)}$$

$$= \frac{75\ mL \times 60}{20\ min}$$

$$= 225\ mL/h$$

Exercise 4C *Each of the following medications has been added to a burette. Calculate the required pump setting in mL/h for the given infusion time. Give answers to the nearest whole number.*

	Medication	*Infusion time*
1	40 mL of fluid containing 600 mg of penicillin	20 minutes
2	120 mL of fluid containing 500 mg of vancomycin	50 minutes
3	100 mL of fluid containing 1 g of flucloxacillin	30 minutes
4	50 mL of fluid containing 0.5 g of potassium chloride	half an hour
5	60 mL of fluid containing 75 mg of ranitidine	35 minutes
6	80 mL of fluid containing 80 mg of gentamicin	45 minutes
7	75 mL of fluid containing 75 mg of gentamicin	40 minutes
8	70 mL of fluid containing 1.2 g of penicillin	25 minutes

Example 5 *750 mL of fluid is to be given over 5 hours. The I.V. set delivers 20 drops per millilitre. At what rate (in drops per minute) should it drip?*

$$\text{Rate (drops/min)} = \frac{\text{Volume (drops)}}{\text{Time (minutes)}}$$

$$= \frac{\text{Volume (drops)}}{\text{Time (hours)} \times 60}$$

$$= \frac{750 \text{ mL} \times 20 \text{ drops/mL}}{5 \text{ h} \times 60}$$

$$= \frac{750 \times 20 \text{ drops}}{5 \times 60 \text{ min}}$$

$$= \frac{750}{5} \times \frac{1}{3} \text{ drops/min} \qquad \left[\text{since } \frac{20}{60} = \frac{1}{3}\right]$$

$$= \frac{150}{3} \text{ drops/min} \qquad \left[\text{since } \frac{750}{5} = 150\right]$$

$$= 50 \text{ drops/min}$$

Example 6 *A patient is to receive half a litre of dextrose 5% over 4 hours. The giving set delivers 20 drops/mL. Calculate the required drip rate in drops/min. Give the answer to the nearest whole number.*

$$\text{Half a litre} = 500 \text{ mL}$$

$$\text{Rate (drops/min)} = \frac{\text{Volume (drops)}}{\text{Time (minutes)}}$$

$$= \frac{\text{Volume (drops)}}{\text{Time (hours)} \times 60}$$

$$= \frac{500 \text{ mL} \times 20 \text{ drops/mL}}{4 \text{ h} \times 60}$$

$$= \frac{500 \times 20 \text{ drops}}{4 \times 60 \text{ min}}$$

$$= \frac{500}{4} \times \frac{1}{3} \text{ drops/min} \qquad \left[\text{since } \frac{20}{60} = \frac{1}{3}\right]$$

$$= \frac{125}{3} \text{ drops/min} \qquad \left[\text{since } \frac{500}{5} = 125\right]$$

$$\Rightarrow 42 \text{ drops/min}$$
(to nearest whole number)

$$3\overline{)125.^20}$$
$$41.\textcircled{6}$$

Exercise 4D *Calculate the required drip rate in drops per minute.*
Give each answer to the nearest whole number.

1   An infant is ordered 150 mL of Hartmann's solution to run over
    6 hours. The microdrip delivers 60 drops per millilitre.

2   A teenager is to receive 500 mL of dextrose 5% over 8 hours.
    The I.V. set emits 20 drops/mL.

3   0.5 litre of dextrose 4% in $\frac{1}{5}$ normal saline is to run over
    12 hours. The administration set delivers 20 drops/mL.

4   750 mL of normal saline is to be given to a patient over 9 hours
    using a giving set which emits 20 drops/mL.

5   An adult male is to be given half a litre of normal saline over
    5 hours using an I.V. set which gives 20 drops per millilitre.

6   A female patient is to receive $1\frac{1}{2}$ litres of fluid over 10 hours.
    The giving set delivers 20 drops/mL.

7   A patient is to have the remaining 300 mL of dextrose 5% run
    through in 50 minutes. The administration set gives 20
    drops/mL.

8   400 mL of normal saline is to be infused over 10 hours using a
    microdrop giving set. The set delivers 60 drops/mL.

9   A child is ordered 24 mL/h of normal saline. The microdrop
    delivers 60 drops/mL.

    Note: 24 mL/h = 24 mL in one hour

Example 7 *One unit of packed cells is to be run over 2 hours. The unit of packed cells contains 250 mL. The I.V. set to be used emits 20 drops/mL. Calculate the drip rate in drops/min. Give the answer to the nearest whole number.*

$$\text{Rate (drops/min)} = \frac{\text{Volume (drops)}}{\text{Time (minutes)}}$$

$$= \frac{\text{Volume (drops)}}{\text{Time (hours)} \times 60}$$

$$= \frac{250 \text{ mL} \times 20 \text{ drops/mL}}{2 \text{ h} \times 60}$$

$$= \frac{250 \times 20 \text{ drops}}{2 \times 60 \text{ min}}$$

$$= \frac{250}{2} \times \frac{1}{3} \text{ drops/min} \quad \left[\text{since } \frac{20}{60} = \frac{1}{3}\right]$$

$$= \frac{125}{3} \text{ drops/min}$$

$$\Rightarrow 42 \text{ drops/min}$$

$$3 \overline{)125.\overset{2}{0}}$$
$$41.\enclose{circle}{6}$$

Exercise 4E *Calculate the drip rate in drops per minute for each of the following blood infusions. Give each answer to the nearest whole number.*

1 An anaemic patient must be given one unit of packed cells over 4 hours. The unit of packed cells holds 250 mL.
The I.V. set delivers 20 drops per mL.

2 A postoperative adult male is to be given one unit of autologous blood in 4 hours.
The unit of autologous blood has a volume of 500 mL.
The giving set emits 20 drops/mL.

3 Towards the end of a transfusion, the doctor orders that the remaining half unit of packed cells is to be administered over one hour. A full unit of packed cells is 250 mL. The I.V. giving set delivers 20 drops per mL.

4 300 mL of autologous blood is to be transfused over 2 hours using an administration set which gives 20 drops per mL.

5 One unit of packed red cells is to be run over 3 hours. The unit of packed cells contains 350 mL. An I.V. set which emits 15 drops/mL is to be used.

6 A patient is to be given one unit of autologous blood over 3 hours using a giving set which delivers 15 drops/mL. The unit of blood contains 480 mL.

7 An administration set which emits 15 drops/mL is to be used to give a 480 mL unit of autologous blood over $3\frac{1}{2}$ hours.

8 A 350 mL unit of packed cells is to be run over $2\frac{1}{2}$ hours using an I.V. giving set which delivers 15 drops/mL.

Example 8 *At 0730 hours, a 500 mL flask of normal saline is set up to run at 80 mL/h. At what time would the flask have to be replaced?*

$$\text{Running time (hours)} = \frac{\text{Volume (mL)}}{\text{Rate (mL/h)}}$$

$$= \frac{500 \text{ mL}}{80 \text{ mL/h}}$$

$$= 6\tfrac{1}{4} \text{ h or 6 h 15 min}$$

$$\therefore \text{ Finishing time } = 0730 \text{ h} + 6 \text{ h } 15 \text{ min} = 1345 \text{ hours}$$

Example 9 *At 0600 hours, a one litre flask of normal saline is set up to run through an infusion pump at 70 mL/h. After 8 hours, the flow rate is increased to 80 mL/h. By what time would the flask have to be replaced?*

i Volume (mL) $= \text{Rate (mL/h)} \times \text{Time (h)}$

$= 70 \text{ mL/h} \times 8 \text{ h}$

$= 560 \text{ mL}$

ii One litre $= 1000 \text{ mL}$

$\therefore$ Volume remaining $= 1000\text{mL} - 560 \text{ mL} = 440 \text{ mL}$

iii Running time (hours) $= \dfrac{\text{Volume (mL)}}{\text{Rate (mL/h)}}$

$= \dfrac{440 \text{ mL}}{80 \text{ mL/h}}$

$= 5\tfrac{1}{2} \text{ h or 5 h 30 min}$

iv Total running time $= 8 \text{ h} + 5\tfrac{1}{2} \text{ h} = 13\tfrac{1}{2} \text{ h or 13 h 30 min}$

v $\therefore$ Finishing time $= 0600 \text{ h} + 13 \text{ h } 30 \text{ min} = 1930 \text{ hours}$

Exercise 4F

1 A patient has *two* intravenous lines inserted. One line is running at 45 mL/h; the other at 30 mL/h. What volume of fluid would this patient receive in a 24-hour period?

2 At 0800 h, one litre of dextrose 4% and $\frac{1}{5}$ normal saline is set up to run at 75 mL/h. At what time would the flask be finished?

3 At 2100 hours on a Monday, one litre of dextrose 5% is set up to run at 50 mL/h. When will the flask be finished?

4 One litre of Hartmann's solution is to be given I.V. For the first 6 hours the solution is delivered at 85 mL/h, then the rate is reduced to 70 mL/h. Find the total time taken to give the full volume.

5 A patient is to receive half a litre of dextrose 5% I.V. A flask is set up at 0800 hours running at 60 mL/h. After 5 hours the rate is increased to 80 mL/h. At what time will the I.V. be completed?

6 At 0430 hours, an infusion pump is set to deliver 1.5 litres of fluid at a rate of 90 mL/h. After 10 hours the pump is reset to 75 mL/h. Calculate the finishing time.

7 A one litre I.V. flask of normal saline has been running for 6 hours at a rate of 75 mL/h. The doctor orders the remaining contents to be run through in the next 5 hours. Calculate the new flow rate.

8 A patient is to receive one litre of dextrose 4% in $\frac{1}{5}$ normal saline.
For the first $3\frac{1}{2}$ hours the fluid is delivered at 160 mL/h.
A specialist then orders the rate slowed so that the remaining fluid will be run over the next 8 hours. Calculate the required flow rate.

$$\frac{\text{Concentration of}}{\text{stock (mg/mL)}} = \frac{\text{Stock strength (mg)}}{\text{Volume of stock solution (mL)}}$$

$$\text{then: Dosage (mg/h)} = \text{Rate (mL/h)} \times \text{Concentration of stock (mg/mL)}$$

$$\text{and: Rate (mL/h)} = \frac{\text{Dosage (mg/h)}}{\text{Concentration of stock (mg/mL)}}$$

Example 10 *A young postoperative patient's I.V. analgesic order is for pethidine 300 mg in 500 mL of normal saline. The solution is to run at between 10 and 40 mL/h, depending on the nurse's assessment of pain. a Calculate the concentration of the pethidine/saline solution. b How many milligrams of pethidine will the patient receive each hour if the infusion is run at 25 mL/h? c At what rate (in mL/h) should the nurse set the pump to administer the pethidine at 8 mg/h?*

a Concentration $= \dfrac{300 \text{ mg}}{500 \text{ mL}} = \dfrac{3}{5}$ mg/mL or 0.6 mg/mL

b Dosage $= 25 \text{ mL/h} \times 0.6 \text{ mg/mL} = 15 \text{ mg/h}$

c Rate $= \dfrac{8 \text{ mg/h}}{0.6 \text{ mg/mL}} = \dfrac{80}{6}$ mL/h $= 13.3 \Rightarrow 13$ mL/h

$$6 \overline{)8^{2}0.^{2}0}$$
$$13.\textcircled{3}$$

Example 11 *A postoperative female patient has a patient controlled analgesia (PCA) running. The flask contains morphine 50 mg in 100 mL of normal saline. The PCA has been set, as per doctor's orders, so that when the patient presses the button she receives a bolus dose of 1 mL. a Calculate the concentration of the morphine/saline solution. b How much morphine does the bolus dose contain?*

a Concentration $= \dfrac{50 \text{ mg}}{100 \text{ mL}} = \dfrac{1}{2}$ mg/mL or 0.5 mg/mL

b Dosage (mg) $= \text{Volume (mL)} \times \text{Concentration of stock (mg/mL)}$
$\therefore$ Dosage $= 1 \text{ mL} \times 0.5 \text{ mg/mL} = 0.5 \text{ mg}$

Exercise 4G

1 A young postoperative patient is ordered pethidine 350 mg in 500 mL of normal saline. The solution is to run at between 10 and 40 mL/h, depending on the nurse's assessment of pain.

  a What is the concentration (mg/mL) of the pethidine/saline solution?

  b How many milligrams of pethidine will the patient receive hourly if the infusion is run at   **i** 10 mL/h   **ii** 15 mL/h   **iii** 25 mL/h   **iv** 40 mL/h?

  c At what rate (mL/h) should the pump be set to deliver the pethidine at   **i** 9 mg/h   **ii** 12 mg/h   **iii** 20 mg/h   **iv** 25 mg/h?
    [Give each answer to nearest whole number.]

2 An adult male patient is ordered morphine 50 mg in 500 mL of normal saline. The solution is to be infused at 10–40 mL/h using a volumetric infusion pump.

  a Calculate the concentration (mg/mL) of the morphine/saline solution.

  b How many milligrams of morphine will the patient receive per hour if the pump is set at   **i** 10 mL/h   **ii** 15 mL/h   **iii** 20 mL/h   **iv** 40 mL/h?

  c At what rate (mL/h) should the pump be set to deliver the morphine at   **i** 1.5 mg/h   **ii** 2.5 mg/h   **iii** 3 mg/h   **iv** 3.5 mg/h?

3 A postoperative patient has a patient controlled analgesia (PCA) infusion running via a syringe pump. The syringe contains fentanyl 300 mcg in 30 mL of normal saline. The PCA has been set, in accordance with doctor's orders, so that when the button is pressed the patient receives a bolus dose of 1 mL.

  a What is the concentration (mcg/mL) of the solution in the syringe?

  b How much fentanyl is in each bolus dose?

  c If the patient has six bolus doses within an hour, how much fentanyl has the patient received in that hour?

Example 12 *One gram of dextrose provides 16 kilojoules of energy. How many kilojoules does a patient receive from an infusion of $1\frac{1}{2}$ litres of 10% dextrose?*

10% dextrose	=	10 g of dextrose per 100 mL of solution
	=	$\dfrac{10 \text{ g}}{100 \text{ mL}}$
$1\frac{1}{2}$ litres	=	1500 mL
Weight of dextrose	=	Volume of infusion $\times$ strength of solution
	=	$\dfrac{1500 \text{ mL} \times 10 \text{ g}}{100 \text{ mL}}$
	=	15×10 g $[1500 \text{ mL} \div 100 \text{ mL} = 15]$
	=	150 g
Energy supplied	=	$150 \text{ g} \times 16 \text{ kJ/g}$
	=	2400 kJ

The symbol for kilojoules is kJ.

Note: The given percentage of dextrose is equal to the number of grams of dextrose per 100 mL of solution.

For example:
5% dextrose = 5 g of dextrose per 100 mL of solution
10% dextrose = 10 g of dextrose per 100 mL of solution
25% dextrose = 25 g of dextrose per 100 mL of solution
50% dextrose = 50 g of dextrose per 100 mL of solution

Exercise 4H *One gram of carbohydrate provides 16 kilojoules of energy. Dextrose and glucose are carbohydrates. Calculate how many kilojoules are supplied to a patient in each of the following infusions.*

1   1 L of 5% dextrose

2 $2\frac{1}{2}$ L of 5% dextrose

3   1 L of 10% dextrose

4   500 mL of 25% dextrose

5   2 L of normal saline
       Normal saline is a 0.9% solution of salt in water.

6   750 mL of 4% dextrose in $\frac{1}{5}$ normal saline

7 $1\frac{1}{2}$ L of Hartmann's solution
       Hartmann's solution contains sodium lactate, sodium chloride, potassium chloride, and calcium chloride.

8   A diabetic patient is found unconscious and presumed to be hypoglycaemic. 50 mL of 50% glucose is given to the patient. How many kilojoules of energy are administered in the 50 mL dose?

CHAPTER 4 Revision

1 A male patient is receiving dextrose 5% at a rate of 55 mL/h. How much fluid will he receive in
a 2 h **b** 5 h **c** 11 h?

2 A patient is to receive one litre of Hartmann's solution. If an infusion pump is set at 120 mL/h, how long will the pump take to give the solution?

3 1.5 litres of dextrose 4% in $\frac{1}{5}$ normal saline is to be given to a patient over 20 hours. Calculate the required flow rate setting for a volumetric infusion pump.

4 An infusion pump is to be used to give one litre of fluid over 11 hours. At what flow rate should the pump be set?

5 100 mL of fluid containing vancomycin 400 mg has been added to a burette. The infusion is to be given over 45 minutes. Calculate the required pump setting in mL/h, to the nearest whole number.

6 600 mL of normal saline is to be infused over 12 hours using a microdrop giving set. The set delivers 60 drops per millilitre. Calculate the required drip rate in drops per minute.

7 One unit of packed cells is to be given to a patient over 3 hours. The giving set delivers 20 drops/mL. Calculate the drip rate in drops/min if one unit of packed cells contains 250 mL. Give the answer to the nearest whole number.

8 A patient is to be given $1\frac{1}{2}$ litres of fluid over 10 hours. The giving set emits 20 drops/mL. Calculate the required drip rate in drops/min.

9 A female patient is to receive one litre of Hartmann's solution over 12 hours. Calculate the drip rate if the administration set gives 15 drops/mL.

10 A patient is receiving fluid from *two* I.V. lines. One line is running at 65 mL/h; the other at 70 mL/h. What volume of fluid would the patient receive I.V. over 12 hours?

11 At 0700 hours, half a litre of dextrose 5% is set up to run at 40 mL/h. At what time will the flask be finished?

12 A litre of dextrose 5% is to be given I.V. The solution is to run at 75 mL/h for the first 6 hours, then the rate is to be reduced to 50 mL/h. Calculate the *total* time required to give the full volume.

13 At 0300 hours, 2 L of normal saline is set running through an infusion pump at 85 mL/h. After 8 hours the rate is increased to 120 mL/h. Calculate the finishing time.

14 A one litre I.V. flask of normal saline has been running at 90 mL/h for 6 hours. A specialist then orders the rate to be increased so that the remaining solution will be run through in the next 4 hours. Calculate the new flow rate in mL/h.

15 A postoperative patient is ordered morphine 25 mg in 50 mL of normal saline via an infusion pump. **a** Calculate the concentration (mg/mL) of the morphine/saline solution. **b** How many milligrams of morphine will the patient receive hourly if the pump is set at 5 mL/h? **c** At what rate (mL/h) should the pump be set to deliver morphine at 3.5 mg/h?

16 A postoperative patient is receiving a PCA infusion of fentanyl 250 mcg in 25 mL of normal saline via a syringe pump. The PCA is set to give a bolus dose of 1 mL each time the button is pressed. **a** What is the concentration (mcg/mL) of the fentanyl/saline solution? **b** How much fentanyl is in each bolus dose? **c** If the patient has five bolus doses between 1400 hours and 1500 hours on a Sunday, how much fentanyl has the patient received in that hour?

17 One gram of dextrose provides 16 kJ of energy. How many kilojoules does a patient receive from an infusion of 1.5 L of 5% dextrose?

5. Paediatric dosages

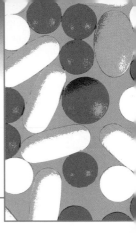

Children grow at different rates.

Most drug dosages are based on the body weight of the infant or child. However, for certain drugs, the dosages are based on body surface area (see pages 102-107).

Great care must be taken when administering drugs to children: *the smallest error is potentially life-threatening.*

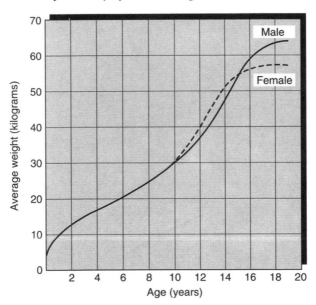

Fig. 5.1 Age and average weight of males and females.
There are wide variations from these averages. Consequently, dosages are based on actual body weight.

Example 1 *A child is prescribed erythromycin. The recommended dosage is 40 mg/kg/day, 4 doses daily. If the child's weight is 15 kg, calculate the size of a single dose.*

```
     15  kg
  ×  40  mg/kg/day
 4)600   mg/day
    150   mg/dose
```

Example 2 *A child is to be given ampicillin. The recommended dosage is 80 mg/kg/day, 4 doses per day. Calculate the size of a single dose if the child's weight is 27 kg.*

```
     27  kg
  ×  80  mg/kg/day
 4)2160  mg/day
    540   mg/dose
```

Exercise 5A *Calculate single doses according to each child's body weight.*

Calculate the size of a single dose for a child weighing 12 kg:

1 Erythromycin, 40 mg/kg/day, 4 doses per day

2 Penicillin V, 50 mg/kg/day, 4 doses per day

3 Cefalexin, 30 mg/kg/day, 4 doses per day

Calculate the size of a single dose for a child weighing 20 kg:

4 Cloxacillin, 50 mg/kg/day, 4 doses per day

5 Chloramphenicol, 40 mg/kg/day, 4 doses per day

6 Amoxicillin, 45 mg/kg/day, 4 doses per day

Calculate the size of a single dose for a child weighing 36 kg:

7 Flucloxacillin, 100 mg/kg/day, 4 doses per day

8 Capreomycin sulphate, 20 mg/kg/day, 3 doses per day

9 Cephalothin, 60 mg/kg/day, 4 doses per day

Example 3 *A boy is ordered pethidine 35 mg, I.M. Stock ampoules contain 50 mg in 1 mL. What volume must be withdrawn for injection?*

$$\begin{aligned} \text{Volume required} &= \frac{\text{Strength required}}{\text{Stock strength}} \times \left[\begin{array}{c} \text{Volume of} \\ \text{stock solution} \end{array} \right] \\ &= \frac{35 \text{ mg}}{50 \text{ mg}} \times 1 \text{ mL} \\ &= \frac{7}{10} \text{ mL or } 0.7 \text{ mL} \end{aligned}$$

Example 4 *A child is ordered digoxin 40 micrograms, I.V. Paediatric ampoules contain 50 mcg/2 mL. Calculate the amount to be drawn up.*

$$\begin{aligned} \text{Volume required} &= \frac{\text{Strength required}}{\text{Stock strength}} \times \left[\begin{array}{c} \text{Volume of} \\ \text{stock solution} \end{array} \right] \\ &= \frac{40 \text{ mcg}}{50 \text{ mcg}} \times 2 \text{ mL} \\ &= \frac{8}{5} \text{ mL or } 1.6 \text{ mL} \end{aligned}$$

Example 5 *A child is to be given 125 mg of capreomycin sulphate. Stock on hand has a strength of 1 g in 2 mL. What volume of stock must be injected?*

$$\begin{aligned} \text{Volume required} &= \frac{\text{Strength required}}{\text{Stock strength}} \times \left[\begin{array}{c} \text{Volume of} \\ \text{stock solution} \end{array} \right] \\ &= \frac{125 \text{ mg}}{1000 \text{ mg}} \times 2 \text{ mL} \quad [1 \text{ g} = 1000 \text{ mg}] \\ &= \frac{25}{100} \text{ mL or } 0.25 \text{ mL} \end{aligned}$$

Exercise 5B *Calculate the volume to be withdrawn for injection for each of these paediatric dosages.*

	Ordered		Stock
1	Pethidine	20 mg	50 mg in 1 mL
2	Pethidine	10 mg	25 mg in 1 mL
3	Metoclopramide	4 mg	10 mg in 2 mL
4	Atropine	0.3 mg	0.4 mg in 1 mL
5	Digoxin	125 mcg	0.5 mg/2 mL
6	Digoxin	18 μg	50 μg in 2 mL
7	Capreomycin sulphate	200 mg	1 g in 2 mL
8	Capreomycin sulphate	150 mg	1 g in 5 mL
9	Cephalothin	120 mg	500 mg in 2 mL
10	Cephalothin	300 mg	500 mg in 2 mL
11	Flucloxacillin	400 mg	1 g in 3 mL
12	Flucloxacillin	100 mg	1 g in 3 mL
13	Phenobarbitone	50 mg	200 mg/mL
14	Aminophylline	180 mg	250 mg in 10 mL
15	Morphine	6.5 mg	10 mg in 1 mL
16	Gentamicin	15 mg	20 mg/2 mL
17	Gentamicin	40 mg	60 mg/1.5 mL
18	Morphine	8 mg	10 mg/mL
19	Furosemide (frusemide)	4.5 mg	20 mg in 2 mL
20	Omnopon	16 mg	20 mg per mL
21	Naloxone	0.03 mg	0.02 mg/mL
22	Naloxone	0.05 mg	0.02 mg/mL

Check that each answer makes sense. Is the volume to be drawn up equal to, less than, or more than the volume of the stock ampoule?

Check your answers on p 134

Example 6 *A child is ordered 80 mg of paracetamol elixir. Stock on hand is 100 mg in 5 mL. Calculate the volume to be given.*

$$\begin{aligned} \text{Volume required} &= \frac{\text{Strength required}}{\text{Stock strength}} \times \left[\text{Volume of stock solution} \right] \\ &= \frac{80 \text{ mg}}{100 \text{ mg}} \times 5 \text{ mL} \\ &= 4 \text{ mL} \end{aligned}$$

Example 7 *A child is to be given 175 micrograms of digoxin, orally. Paediatric mixture contains 50 mcg per mL. Calculate the required volume.*

$$\begin{aligned} \text{Volume required} &= \frac{\text{Strength required}}{\text{Stock strength}} \times \left[\text{Volume of stock solution} \right] \\ &= \frac{175 \text{ mcg}}{50 \text{ mcg}} \times 1 \text{ mL} \\ &= \frac{7}{2} \text{ mL or 3.5 mL} \end{aligned}$$

Example 8 *A child is prescribed 180 mg of flucloxacillin. On hand is stock containing 150 mg in 5 mL. How much should be given?*

$$\begin{aligned} \text{Volume required} &= \frac{\text{Strength required}}{\text{Stock strength}} \times \left[\text{Volume of stock solution} \right] \\ &= \frac{180 \text{ mg}}{150 \text{ mg}} \times 5 \text{ mL} \\ &= 6 \text{ mL} \end{aligned}$$

Exercise 5C *Calculate the volume to be given orally for these paediatric dosages. (The strength of the stock is given in brackets.)*

1 70 mg of paracetamol elixir
  (100 mg/5 mL)

2 300 mg of paracetamol elixir
  (120 mg/5 mL)

3 12.5 mg of promethazine elixir
  (5 mg/5 mL)

4 70 mg of theophylline syrup
  (50 mg/5 mL)

5 125 mcg of digoxin elixir
  (50 mcg/mL)

6 24 mg of phenytoin suspension
  (30 mg/5 mL)

7 200 mg of penicillin suspension
  (125 mg/5 mL)

8 350 mg of penicillin suspension
  (125 mg/5 mL)

9 60 mg of theophylline syrup
  (80 mg/15 mL)

10 225 mg of amoxicillin syrup
  (1 g/10 mL)

11 1.5 mg of clonazepam syrup
  (2.5 mg/mL)

12 50 mg of amoxicillin syrup
  (1 g/10 mL)

13 100 mg of flucloxacillin syrup
  (125 mg/5 mL)

Drugs in powder form

Some medications are supplied in vials containing the drug in powder form. When a known volume of water-for-injection (WFI) is mixed with the vial of powder, the resulting solution has a volume greater than the volume of the WFI. The concentration of the solution (mg/mL) depends upon the volume of WFI used. Some drug labels show the various amounts of WFI to be added to the vial to yield given concentrations of solutions.

Example 9 *Stock vial: benzylpenicillin 600 mg*

For concentration of:	150	200	300	*mg/mL*
Add:	3.6	2.6	1.6	*mL of WFI*

A 12 kg child is ordered 270 mg of benzylpenicillin to be given 8 hourly I.V. How much solution should be drawn up for injection if the concentration, after dilution with WFI, is   (a) 150 mg/mL (b) 200 mg/mL   (c) 300 mg/mL?

$$\frac{\text{Volume}}{\text{required}} = \frac{\text{Strength required}}{\text{Stock strength}} \times \left[\begin{array}{c}\text{Volume of}\\ \text{stock solution}\end{array}\right]$$

a $\dfrac{\text{Volume}}{\text{required}} = \dfrac{270 \text{ mg}}{150 \text{ mg}} \times 1 \text{ mL}$

$= \dfrac{9}{5} \text{ mL}$

$= 1.8 \text{ mL}$

$$5\overline{)9.\overset{4}{0}}$$
$$\underline{1.8}$$

b $\dfrac{\text{Volume}}{\text{required}} = \dfrac{270 \text{ mg}}{200 \text{ mg}} \times 1 \text{ mL}$

$= \dfrac{27}{20} \text{ mL}$

$= 1.35 \text{ mL}$

$$10\overline{)27.0}$$
$$2\overline{)2.7\overset{1}{0}}$$
$$\underline{1.35}$$

[This volume could be measured accurately using a 2.5 mL syringe]

c $\dfrac{\text{Volume}}{\text{required}} = \dfrac{270 \text{ mg}}{300 \text{ mg}} \times 1 \text{ mL}$

$= \dfrac{9}{10} \text{ mL}$

$= 0.9 \text{ mL}$

Exercise 5D *WFI stands for water-for-injection.*

1 [Refer to the table in Example 9, on opposite page.]
An 8 kg child is ordered 180 mg of benzylpenicillin, I.V.
How much solution should be drawn up for injection if the
concentration, after dilution with WFI, is **a** 150 mg/mL
b 200 mg/mL **c** 300 mg/mL?

2 *Stock*: amoxicillin 500 mg I.V. vial

For concentration of:	100	125	200	250	mg/mL
Add:	4.6	3.6	2.1	1.6	mL of WFI

Order: amoxicillin 150 mg I.V.

What volume of solution would need to be drawn up for
injection if the concentration, after dilution with WFI, is
a 100 mg/mL **b** 125 mg/mL **c** 200 mg/mL **d** 250 mg/mL?

3 *Label*: Ampicillin 500 mg multiple dose vial.
Reconstitution: Add 1.8 mL of WFI to yield 250 mg/mL.
What volume of the reconstituted mixture should be drawn up
for injection if the order is for **a** 100 mg **b** 150 mg
c 200 mg of ampicillin?

4 *Label on vial*: Keflin 1 gram
Reconstitution: Add 4 mL of WFI to yield 0.5 g/2.2 mL.
Calculate the volume of reconstituted mixture to be drawn up
for injection if the order is for **a** 200 mg **b** 300 mg
c 350 mg of keflin.

Give answers greater than 1 mL correct to one decimal place;
answers less than 1 mL correct to two decimal places.

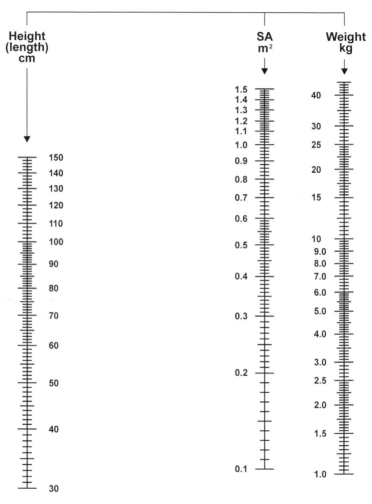

Fig. 5.2 Nomogram for calculating body surface area. Body surface area (SA) is shown when height (or length) and weight are linked by a straight edge (use a ruler).

Calculations of paediatric dosages based on body surface area

As mentioned previously, the dosages for the administration of drugs to paediatric patients may be based on *body surface area*. An example is in the administration of cytotoxic drugs as these drugs can have severe side effects. Body surface area is a major factor in heat loss and moisture loss from the body.

The nomogram (Fig. 5.2 on the opposite page) is a graph that relates a person's height (or length), weight and body surface area. Once the height (length) and weight of a patient have been measured then the body surface area can be determined using the nomogram.

For example, if a child has a height of 85 cm and a weight of 15 kg, then the child's body surface area is found by linking the height and weight measurements with a straight edge: the area is 0.61 m^2.

SA on the nomogram stands for *body surface area*.

Children of the same age have a wide range of heights (lengths) and weights and, consequently, a wide range of body surface areas.

Example 10 *Using the nomogram on page 102, find the body surface area of a 6-month-old infant with a length of 65 cm and weight of 8.2 kg.*

On the nomogram, join length 65 cm and weight 8.2 kg with a straight edge (e.g. ruler). The straight edge then crosses the body surface area scale (marked SA) at 0.40 m^2.

Example 11 *Using the nomogram, determine the body surface area of a 2-year-old boy of height 87 cm and weight 13.5 kg.*

On the nomogram, join height 87 cm and weight 13.5 kg with a straight edge. The straight edge then crosses the body surface area scale at 0.58 m^2.

Exercise 5E *The lengths (heights) and weights used below represent children from 3 months to 3 years of age. Use the nomogram to find the body surface area of each child. Estimate answers to the nearest 0.01 m²*

1 **a** Length 65 cm, weight 6.4 kg
   b Length 65 cm, weight 8.2 kg

2 **a** Length 73 cm, weight 8.8 kg
   b Length 73 cm, weight 10.5 kg

3 **a** Length 85 cm, weight 11.0 kg
   b Length 85 cm, weight 13.5 kg

4 **a** Height 94 cm, weight 12.5 kg
   b Height 94 cm, weight 15.5 kg

5 **a** Weight 5.7 kg, length 57 cm
   b Weight 5.7 kg, length 63 cm

6 **a** Weight 9.4 kg, length 68 cm
   b Weight 9.4 kg, length 74 cm

7 **a** Weight 11.5 kg, length 78 cm
   b Weight 11.5 kg, length 86 cm

8 **a** Weight 14.0 kg, height 87 cm
   b Weight 14.0 kg, height 97 cm

9 **a** Length 67 cm, weight 10.0 kg
   b Length 78 cm, weight 9.0 kg

10 **a** Weight 13.0 kg, height 90 cm
   b Weight 14.0 kg, height 81 cm

Example 12 *A young patient with leukaemia is to be given his weekly injection of doxorubicin. The recommended dosage is 30 mg/m² and the boy's body surface area has been determined at 0.48 m². Stock solution contains doxorubicin 10 mg/5 mL. Calculate volume to be drawn up for injection.*

0.48	m²	Body surface area
× 30	mg/m²	Recommended dosage
14.40	mg	Dose required

$$\frac{\text{Volume}}{\text{required}} = \frac{\text{Strength required}}{\text{Stock strength}} \times \begin{bmatrix} \text{Volume of} \\ \text{stock solution} \end{bmatrix}$$

$$= \frac{14.4 \text{ mg}}{10 \text{ mg}} \times 5 \text{ mL}$$

$$= 7.2 \text{ mL}$$

Exercise 5F *The aim of this exercise is to introduce the method of calculating drug doses based on body surface areas. These doses are used in complex situations, such as the treatment of children with leukaemia, and are administered under very strict procedures and supervision. Calculate the volume required in each case.*

1 *Prescribed*: dactinomycin
   Recommended dosage: 1.5 mg/m^2
   Stock strength: 500 mcg/mL
   Body surface area: 0.40 m^2

2 *Prescribed*: bleomycin
   Recommended dosage: 10 units/m^2
   Stock strength: 15 units/5 mL
   Body surface area: 0.54 m^2

3 *Prescribed*: cytarabine
   Recommended dosage: 120 mg/m^2
   Stock strength: 100 mg/5 mL
   Body surface area: 0.45 m^2

4 *Prescribed*: daunorubicin
   Recommended dosage: 30 mg/m^2
   Stock strength: 20 mg/5 mL
   Body surface area: 0.52 m^2

5 *Prescribed*: vincristine
   Recommended dosage: 1.5 mg/m^2
   Stock strength: 1 mg/mL
   Body surface area: 0.64 m^2

6 *Prescribed*: cyclophosphamide
   Recommended dosage: 1000 mg/m^2
   Stock strength: 1 g/50mL
   Body surface area: 0.57 m^2

CHAPTER 5 Revision

1 A child is prescribed cloxacillin. The recommended dosage is 50 mg/kg/day, 4 doses daily. Calculate the size of a *single* dose if the child's weight is 22 kg.

2 A young boy weighing 19 kg is to be given cephalothin. The recommended dosage is 60 mg/kg/day, 4 doses daily. What should be the size of a *single* dose?

3 The recommended dosage for capreomycin sulphate is 20 mg/kg/day, 3 doses daily. Calculate the size of a *single* dose for a girl weighing 27 kg.

4 A girl is ordered pethidine 15 mg. Stock ampoules on hand contain 50 mg in 2 mL. What volume must be withdrawn for injection?

5 A child is prescribed amoxicillin 320 mg. Stock contains 1 g in 3 mL. What volume should be injected?

6 An injection of morphine 4 mg is to be given. Calculate the amount to be drawn up if ampoules contain 10 mg/1.5 mL.

7 A child is to be given 180 mg of paracetamol. Stock elixir contains 120 mg/5 mL. Calculate the volume to be given orally.

8 A boy is prescribed clonazepam 1.8 mg, to be taken orally. What volume of syrup should be given if stock contains 2.5 mg/mL?

9 A young patient is ordered penicillin 300 mg. The suspension on hand has a strength of 125 mg/5 mL. How much suspension should be given?

10 A girl is to receive amoxicillin 160 mg, I.V. What volume of solution should be drawn up for injection if the concentration, after dilution with water-for-injection, is: **a** 100 mg/mL **b** 200 mg/mL **c** 250 mg/mL?

11 A vial of ampicillin 500 mg is reconstituted with 1.8 mL of water-for-injection to give a concentration of 250 mg/mL. Calculate the volume of this solution that should be drawn up for injection if the order is for **a** 75 mg   **b** 80 mg **c** 175 mg   **d** 180 mg

Use the nomogram on page 102 to work out the answers to questions 12–15:

12 Find the body surface area of a 4-year-old girl of height 102 cm and weight 16.5 kg.

13 A 5-year-old boy has a height of 108 cm and he weighs 18.5 kg. Find his body surface area.

14 A girl is 7 years old. Her height is 120 cm and weight 20.5 kg. What is her body surface area?

15 An 8-year-old boy weighs 24 kg and has a height of 124 cm. Determine his body surface area.

16 A boy is to be given bleomycin. The recommended dosage is 10 units per m^2. Reconstituted stock has a strength of 15 units/5 mL. What volume should be injected if the boy has a body surface area of 0.48 m^2?

17 A young patient is prescribed doxorubicin. The recommended dosage is 30 mg/m^2 and stock contains 50 mg/25 mL. Calculate the volume required if the patient's body surface area is 0.70 m^2.

6. Summary exercises

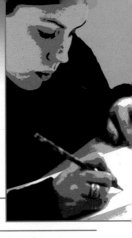

Summary exercise I

1. 450 mg of soluble aspirin is required. Stock on hand is 300 mg tablets. How many tablets should be given?

2. Warfarin tablets are available in strengths of 1 mg, 2 mg, 5 mg, and 10 mg. Choose the best combination of whole tablets for each of the following dosages of warfarin. **a** 4 mg **b** 8 mg **c** 12 mg

3. A solution contains paracetamol 120 mg/5 mL. How many milligrams of paracetamol are in **a** 15 mL **b** 25 mL **c** 40 mL of the solution?

4. A patient is ordered 360 mg of penicillin, orally. The strength of the stock syrup is 125 mg/5 mL. Calculate the volume required.

5. A patient is prescribed benzylpenicillin 1200 mg, I.V. Stock ampoules contain 1 g in 5 mL. Is the volume to be drawn up for injection equal to 5 mL, less than 5 mL, or more than 5 mL?

6. Stock ampoules of erythromycin contain 300 mg/10 mL. Calculate the volume required for injection when a patient is ordered erythromycin 135 mg, I.M.I.

7. 400 mg of benzylpenicillin is to be given I.V. On hand is benzylpenicillin 600 mg in 2 mL. What volume should be drawn up?

Check your answers on p 136

8 A male patient is receiving one litre of dextrose 5% at a rate of 25 mL/h. How much of the solution will he receive over
a 3 h **b** 5 h **c** 12 h?

9 One litre of Hartmann's solution is to be given over 12 hours. Calculate the required flow rate of a volumetric infusion pump.

10 140 mL of fluid containing 600 mg of vancomycin is to be given over 50 minutes. Calculate the required pump setting in mL/h.

11 700 mL of Hartmann's solution is to be given over 8 hours. The I.V. set delivers 20 drops/mL. At what rate should it drip?

12 A patient is to be given one unit of packed cells over 3 hours. Calculate the drip rate in drops/min if the unit of packed cells holds 250 mL and the giving set emits 20 drops per mL. Give the answer to the nearest whole number.

13 800 mL of fluid is to be given I.V. The fluid is run at 70 mL/h for the first 5 hours then the rate is reduced to 60 mL/h. Find the total time taken to give the 800 mL.

14 A patient is ordered pethidine 400 mg in 500 mL of normal saline. The solution is to be infused via an infusion pump at between 10 and 40 mL/h, depending on the nurse's assessment of pain.
a Calculate the concentration of the pethidine/saline solution.
b How many milligrams of pethidine will the patient receive hourly if the pump is run at 15 mL/h?
c At what rate should the pump be set to deliver 20 mg/h? (Give the answer to the nearest whole number.)

15 One gram of dextrose provides 16 kJ of energy. How many kilojoules does a patient receive from an infusion of half a litre of 10% dextrose?

16 A child is prescribed penicillin V. The recommended dosage is 50 mg/kg/day, 4 doses daily. If the child's weight is 18 kg, calculate the size of a single dose.

17 A girl is ordered phenobarbitone 140 mg. Stock ampoules contain 200 mg/mL. What volume must be withdrawn for injection?

18 A child is prescribed 175 mg of capreomycin sulphate by I.M.I. A stock ampoule contains 1 g in 2 mL. What volume of stock should be injected?

19 A young boy is to have 125 mcg of digoxin, orally. Paediatric mixture has a strength of 50 mcg per mL. Calculate the required volume.

20 A young patient is to be given benzylpenicillin 175 mg. What volume of solution should be drawn up for injection if the concentration, after dilution with water-for-injection, is **a** 300 mg/mL   **b** 200 mg/mL   **c** 150 mg/mL?

21 Using the nomogram on page 102, find the body surface area of a 9-month-old girl of length 68 cm and weight 9.2 kg.

22 A child is prescribed dactinomycin I.V. The recommended dosage is 0.9 mg/m^2 and stock on hand has a strength of 500 mcg/mL. Calculate the volume to be injected if the child's body surface area is 0.55 m^2.

Summary exercise II

1 How many 30 mg tablets of phenobarbitone should be given if phenobarbitone 15 mg is prescribed?

2 Thioridazine tablets are available in strengths of 10 mg, 25 mg, 50 mg and 100 mg. What combination of whole tablets should be used for the following dosages **a** 60 mg **b** 85 mg **c** 110 mg?

3 A solution contains fluoxetine 20 mg/5 mL. How many milligrams of fluoxetine are in **a** 15 mL **b** 30 mL **c** 35 mL of the solution?

4 900 mg of benzylpenicillin is to be given orally. Stock mixture contains 250 mg/5 mL. Calculate the volume of mixture to be given.

5 Capreomycin sulphate 900 mg is ordered. Stock ampoules contain 1 g in 3 mL. Is the volume required for injection equal to 3 mL, less than 3 mL, or more than 3 mL?

6 An injection of digoxin 225 mcg is ordered. Stock on hand is digoxin 500 mcg in 2 mL. What volume of stock should be given?

7 A patient is to receive one litre of normal saline, I.V. The infusion pump is set at 80 mL/h. How long will the fluid last?

8 Over the next 9 hours, a patient is to receive half a litre of dextrose 4% in $\frac{1}{5}$ normal saline using a volumetric infusion pump. At what flow rate should the pump be set?

9 150 mL of fluid containing 1.5 g of flucloxacillin is to be infused over 45 minutes. Calculate the required pump setting in mL/h.

10 A child is ordered 120 mL of Hartmann's solution to be given over 5 hours. The microdrip delivers 60 drops/mL. Calculate the required drip rate in drops/min.

Check your answers on p 137

11 A unit of autologous blood is to be given to a patient over 4 hours. The unit of blood contains 480 mL and the giving set delivers 15 drops/mL. Calculate the drip rate in drops/min.

12 At 2200 hours on a Wednesday, one litre of Hartmann's solution is set to run at 80 mL/h. When will the infusion be finished?

13 A patient is to be given 1.2 litres of fluid, I.V. An infusion pump is set at a rate of 60 mL/h. After 12 hours the rate is increased to 96 mL/h. Calculate the total running time.

14 A postoperative patient is to receive a PCA infusion of fentanyl 350 mcg in 35 mL of normal saline, via a syringe pump. The PCA is set to give a bolus dose of 1 mL each time the button is pressed.
  a What is the concentration of the fentanyl/saline solution?
  b How much fentanyl is in each bolus dose?
  c If the patient has four bolus doses between 1100 and 1200 hours on a Friday, how much fentanyl has the patient received in that hour?

15 One gram of dextrose provides 16 kJ of energy. A patient is given an infusion of 2 L of 4% dextrose in $\frac{1}{5}$ normal saline. How many kilojoules does this infusion provide?

16 A child is to be given capreomycin sulphate. The recommended dosage is 20 mg/kg/day, 3 doses per day. Calculate the size of a single dose if the child's weight is 24 kg.

17 It is necessary to give an infant an injection of digoxin 35 micrograms. Paediatric ampoules contain 50 µg/2 mL. Calculate the amount to be drawn up.

18 A boy is ordered 120 mg of paracetamol elixir. Stock on hand has a strength of 100 mg/5 mL. What volume should be given?

19 A young girl is prescribed 700 mg of sulfadiazine, to be taken orally. The stock mixture contains 500 mg/5 mL. How much mixture should be given?

20 A vial of amoxicillin 500 mg is reconstituted with WFI to give a concentration of 200 mg/mL. Calculate the volume of this solution to be drawn up for injection if the order is for
a 50 mg   **b** 90 mg   **c** 120 mg.

21 Using the nomogram on page 102, determine the body surface area of a 2-year-old boy whose height is 87 cm and weight is 13.5 kg.

22 A young girl is to be given cytarabine, I.V. The recommended dosage is 150 mg/m². The girl's body surface area is found to be 0.60 m². Stock on hand has a strength of 500 mg/5 mL. What volume should be drawn up for injection?

7. Answers

Chapter 1: A review of basic calculations

Diagnostic test

1	**a** 830	**b** 8300	**c** 83 000						1A
2	**a** 0.258	**b** 2.58	**c** 25.8						1A
3	**a** 0.378	**b** 0.0378	**c** 0.00378						1B
4	**a** 56.9	**b** 5.69	**c** 0.569						1B
5	**a** 1000	**b** 1000	**c** 1000	**d** 1000					1C
6	**a** 830 g	**b** 6.4 kg							1C
7	**a** 780 mg	**b** 0.034 g							1C
8	**a** 86 micrograms	**b** 0.294 mg							1C
9	**a** 2400 mL	**b** 0.965 L							1C
10	**a** 70 mL	**b** 7 mL	**c** 0.07 L is larger						1D
11	**a** 45 mg	**b** 450 mg	**c** 0.45 g is heavier						1D
12	**a** 27	**b** 2.7	**c** 0.27	**d** 0.0027					1E
13	**a** 468	**b** 4.68	**c** 4.68	**d** 0.468					1E
14	2, 3, 4, 6 and 12 are factors								1F
15	2, 3, 6, 7 and 9 are factors								1F
16	**a** $\frac{2}{3}$	**b** $\frac{7}{9}$							1G
17	**a** $\frac{3}{40}$	**b** $\frac{7}{16}$							1G
18	**a** $\frac{4}{5}$	**b** $\frac{2}{3}$	**c** $\frac{3}{5}$						1H
19	**a** $\frac{7}{10}$	**b** $\frac{4}{5}$	**c** $\frac{2}{5}$						1H
20	**a** $\frac{13}{4}$	**b** $\frac{11}{2}$	**c** $\frac{25}{4}$						1I
21	**a** $\frac{35}{6}$	**b** $\frac{16}{5}$	**c** $\frac{12}{5}$						1I
22	**a** $\frac{2}{3}$	**b** $\frac{9}{10}$	**c** $\frac{400}{9}$	**d** $\frac{9}{5}$					1J

23 **a** 0.7   **b** 1.8   **c** 0.4   *1K*
24 **a** 0.37   **b** 2.63 **c** 0.52   *1K*
25 **a** 1.608   **b** 0.570 **c** 2.657   *1K*
26 **a** 0.625   **b** 0.45 **c** 0.68   **d** 0.775   *1L*
27 **a** 0.2   **b** 0.4   **c** 0.8   *1M*
28 **a** 0.71   **b** 0.56   *1M*
29 **a** 0.233   **b** 0.843   *1M*
30 **a** $31.6 \Rightarrow 32$ **b** $56.2 \Rightarrow 56$ *1N*
31 **a** $9.16 \Rightarrow 9.2$ **b** $7.22 \Rightarrow 7.2$ *1N*
32 **a** $8\frac{1}{2}$ **b** $22\frac{1}{3}$ **c** $22\frac{3}{5}$ *1O*
33 **a** $\frac{11}{4}$ **b** $\frac{77}{6}$ **c** $\frac{142}{5}$ *1O*
34 **a** $\frac{5}{9}$ **b** $1\frac{1}{14}$ **c** $\frac{2}{5}$ *1P*

Exercise 1A   *Multiplication by 10, 100 and 1000*

1 6.8, 68, 680	**9** 0.147, 1.47, 14.7
2 9.75, 97.5, 975	**10** 0.06, 0.6, 6
3 37, 370, 3700	**11** 37.6, 376, 3760
4 56.2, 562, 5620	**12** 6.39, 63.9, 639
5 770, 7700, 77 000	**13** 0.75, 7.5, 75
6 8250, 82 500, 825 000	**14** 0.8, 8, 80
7 2, 20, 200	**15** 0.03, 0.3, 3
8 0.46, 4.6, 46	**16** 0.505, 5.05, 50.5

Exercise 1B   *Division by 10, 100 and 1000*

1 9.84, 0.984, 0.0984	**9** 6.8, 0.68, 0.068
2 0.591, 0.0591, 0.00591	**10** 0.229, 0.0229, 0.00229
3 0.26, 0.026, 0.0026	**11** 5.14, 0.514, 0.0514
4 30.7, 3.07, 0.307	**12** 91.6, 9.16, 0.916
5 8.2, 0.82, 0.082	**13** 6.72, 0.672, 0.0672
6 0.7, 0.07, 0.007	**14** 38.7, 3.87, 0.387
7 0.3, 0.03, 0.003	**15** 0.894, 0.0894, 0.00894
8 0.75, 0.075, 0.0075	**16** 0.0707, 0.00707, 0.000707

Exercise 1C   *Converting metric units*

Grams:

1 5000	**2** 2400	**3** 750	**4** 1625

Kilograms:

5 7	**6** 0.935	**7** 0.085	**8** 0.003

Milligrams:

9 4000	**11** 690	**13** 35	**15** 655
10 8700	**12** 20	**14** 6	**16** 4280

Grams:

17 6	**19** 0.865	**21** 0.07	**23** 0.005
18 7.25	**20** 0.095	**22** 0.002	**24** 0.125

Micrograms:

25	195	27	750	29	80	31	625
26	600	28	75	30	1	32	98

Milligrams:

33	0.825	35	0.065	37	0.01	39	0.2
34	0.75	36	0.095	38	0.005	40	0.03

Millilitres:

41	2000	43	1500	45	1600	47	800
42	30 000	44	4500	46	2240	48	750

Litres:

49	4	51	0.625	53	0.095	55	0.005
50	10	52	0.35	54	0.06	56	0.002

Exercise 1D   *Comparing metric measurements*

1	a	100 mL	b	10 mL	c	0.1 L
2	a	3 mL	b	300 mL	c	0.3 L
3	a	50 mL	b	5 mL	c	0.05 L
4	a	47 mL	b	470 mL	c	0.47 L
5	a	400 mg	b	4 mg	c	0.4 g
6	a	60 mg	b	600 mg	c	0.6 g
7	a	70 mg	b	7 mg	c	0.07 g
8	a	630 mg	b	63 mg	c	0.63 g
9	a	2 mcg	b	20 mcg	c	0.02 mg
10	a	900 mcg	b	90 mcg	c	0.9 mg
11	a	1 mcg	b	100 mcg	c	0.1 mg
12	a	580 mcg	b	58 mcg	c	0.58 mg
13	a	1500 g	b	1050 g	c	1.5 kg
14	a	2080 g	b	2800 g	c	2.8 kg
15	a	950 g	b	95 g	c	0.95 kg
16	a	3350 g	b	3500 g	c	3.5 kg

Exercise 1E *Multiplication of decimals*

1 45, 4.5, 0.45, 0.45
2 14, 0.14, 0.014, 0.0014
3 12, 0.12, 0.12, 0.0012
4 36, 0.36, 0.0036, 0.0036
5 56, 5.6, 0.56, 0.0056
6 102, 10.2, 1.02, 0.102
7 152, 15.2, 0.152, 0.152
8 46, 0.46, 0.046, 0.0046
9 145, 1.45, 1.45, 1.45
10 93, 0.93, 0.0093, 0.093
11 333, 33.3, 0.333, 0.0333
12 287, 0.287, 0.0287, 2.87
13 192, 0.0192, 0.192, 0.0192
14 616, 6.16, 0.0616, 0.616
15 768, 0.768, 0.0768, 0.0768

Exercise 1F *Factors*

1 2, 4, 5
2 3, 4, 12
3 3, 5, 15
4 2, 8, 14
5 3, 4, 12, 15, 20
6 3, 4, 6, 12, 18
7 3, 5, 15, 25
8 5, 17
9 3, 8, 12, 16, 24
10 5, 20, 25
11 4, 9, 12, 18
12 3, 5, 12, 15
13 3, 5, 9, 15
14 4, 8, 12, 16, 18, 24
15 5, 15, 25
16 3, 5, 11, 15
17 5, 7
18 4, 12, 15
19 4, 6, 8, 12, 16
20 6, 14, 15

Exercise 1G *Simplifying fractions I*

Part i

1 $\frac{2}{3}$	**6** $\frac{5}{7}$	**11** $\frac{7}{8}$	**16** $\frac{1}{3}$	**21** $\frac{9}{14}$
2 $\frac{5}{7}$	**7** $\frac{5}{6}$	**12** $\frac{2}{3}$	**17** $\frac{2}{3}$	**22** $\frac{4}{5}$
3 $\frac{3}{8}$	**8** $\frac{4}{5}$	**13** $\frac{3}{7}$	**18** $\frac{7}{8}$	**23** $\frac{13}{16}$
4 $\frac{1}{2}$	**9** $\frac{3}{7}$	**14** $\frac{8}{9}$	**19** $\frac{18}{25}$	**24** $\frac{3}{10}$
5 $\frac{3}{4}$	**10** $\frac{3}{10}$	**15** $\frac{2}{5}$	**20** $\frac{5}{11}$	**25** $\frac{4}{9}$

Part ii

1 $\frac{1}{2}$	**5** $\frac{1}{2}$	**9** $\frac{2}{15}$	**13** $\frac{5}{8}$	**17** $\frac{7}{9}$
2 $\frac{3}{8}$	**6** $\frac{5}{12}$	**10** $\frac{8}{35}$	**14** $\frac{3}{4}$	**18** $\frac{3}{4}$
3 $\frac{3}{10}$	**7** $\frac{5}{16}$	**11** $\frac{3}{10}$	**15** $\frac{11}{16}$	**19** $\frac{17}{24}$
4 $\frac{1}{4}$	**8** $\frac{1}{4}$	**12** $\frac{4}{25}$	**16** $\frac{4}{9}$	**20** $\frac{13}{30}$

Exercise 1H *Simplifying fractions II*

1 $\frac{3}{5}$	**7** $\frac{13}{15}$	**13** $\frac{2}{3}$	**19** $\frac{2}{3}$	**25** $\frac{2}{3}$	**31** $\frac{5}{6}$
2 $\frac{2}{3}$	**8** $\frac{2}{3}$	**14** $\frac{2}{5}$	**20** $\frac{3}{4}$	**26** $\frac{8}{15}$	**32** $\frac{1}{6}$
3 $\frac{3}{4}$	**9** $\frac{2}{5}$	**15** $\frac{9}{10}$	**21** $\frac{9}{10}$	**27** $\frac{5}{6}$	**33** $\frac{3}{20}$
4 $\frac{5}{12}$	**10** $\frac{3}{4}$	**16** $\frac{3}{5}$	**22** $\frac{3}{4}$	**28** $\frac{14}{25}$	**34** $\frac{3}{8}$
5 $\frac{2}{3}$	**11** $\frac{5}{8}$	**17** $\frac{9}{10}$	**23** $\frac{15}{16}$	**29** $\frac{4}{5}$	**35** $\frac{3}{10}$
6 $\frac{5}{6}$	**12** $\frac{3}{8}$	**18** $\frac{6}{25}$	**24** $\frac{2}{5}$	**30** $\frac{7}{10}$	**36** $\frac{11}{16}$

Exercise 1I *Simplifying fractions III*

1 a $\frac{3}{2}$ b $\frac{5}{2}$ c $\frac{15}{4}$ d $\frac{17}{4}$

2 a $\frac{25}{2}$ b $\frac{75}{4}$ c $\frac{75}{2}$ d $\frac{375}{4}$

3 a $\frac{25}{2}$ b $\frac{175}{6}$ c $\frac{125}{3}$ d $\frac{250}{3}$

4 a $\frac{5}{2}$ b $\frac{15}{2}$ c $\frac{19}{2}$ d $\frac{55}{4}$

5 a $\frac{7}{5}$ b $\frac{3}{2}$ c $\frac{12}{5}$ d $\frac{5}{2}$

6 a $\frac{4}{3}$ b $\frac{5}{2}$ c $\frac{25}{2}$ d $\frac{50}{3}$

7 a $\frac{5}{4}$ b $\frac{5}{2}$ c $\frac{55}{8}$ d $\frac{25}{2}$

8 a $\frac{3}{2}$ b $\frac{5}{3}$ c $\frac{5}{2}$ d $\frac{15}{4}$

9 a $\frac{8}{5}$ b $\frac{12}{5}$ c $\frac{32}{5}$ d $\frac{36}{5}$

10 a $\frac{6}{5}$ b $\frac{14}{5}$ c $\frac{22}{5}$ d $\frac{38}{5}$

11 a $\frac{6}{5}$ b $\frac{3}{2}$ c $\frac{8}{3}$ d $\frac{19}{3}$

12 a $\frac{16}{5}$ b $\frac{18}{5}$ c $\frac{24}{5}$ d $\frac{36}{5}$

Exercise 1J *Simplifying fractions IV*

Part i

1 $\frac{4}{5}$	**5** 2	**9** $\frac{5}{2}$	**13** 200	**17** $\frac{5}{4}$
2 $\frac{3}{4}$	**6** $\frac{7}{10}$	**10** $\frac{19}{8}$	**14** $\frac{200}{9}$	**18** $\frac{2}{3}$
3 $\frac{3}{2}$	**7** $\frac{9}{4}$	**11** 80	**15** $\frac{1000}{11}$	**19** 7
4 $\frac{3}{7}$	**8** $\frac{11}{2}$	**12** $\frac{200}{3}$	**16** $\frac{9}{2}$	**20** $\frac{1}{2}$

Part ii

1 $\frac{3}{2}$	**4** $\frac{400}{3}$	**7** 9	**10** $\frac{5}{2}$
2 $\frac{1}{3}$	**5** $\frac{1}{2}$	**8** 120	**11** $\frac{3}{2}$
3 $\frac{3}{4}$	**6** $\frac{3}{4}$	**9** $\frac{5}{8}$	**12** $\frac{200}{7}$

Exercise 1K *Rounding-off decimal numbers*

Part i

1 0.9	**5** 0.6	**9** 2.4	**13** 1.1
2 0.5	**6** 1.0	**10** 1.1	**14** 3.0
3 0.9	**7** 1.6	**11** 0.2	**15** 1.0
4 0.7	**8** 1.2	**12** 2.7	**16** 0.8

Part ii

1 0.33	**5** 0.14	**9** 2.71	**13** 0.63
2 1.67	**6** 0.13	**10** 1.29	**14** 0.78
3 0.88	**7** 0.92	**11** 0.64	**15** 2.43
4 0.83	**8** 1.57	**12** 0.22	**16** 1.86

Part iii

1 0.486	**5** 1.529	**9** 0.816	**13** 3.091
2 0.955	**6** 0.311	**10** 1.120	**14** 0.165
3 0.606	**7** 2.859	**11** 0.165	**15** 2.780
4 1.415	**8** 0.170	**12** 2.963	**16** 1.758

Exercise 1L   *Fraction to a decimal I*

1 0.5	**7** 0.125	**13** 0.04	**19** 0.275
2 0.25	**8** 0.875	**14** 0.32	**20** 0.675
3 0.75	**9** 0.05	**15** 0.68	**21** 0.02
4 0.2	**10** 0.35	**16** 0.88	**22** 0.14
5 0.6	**11** 0.65	**17** 0.025	**23** 0.42
6 0.8	**12** 0.95	**18** 0.225	**24** 0.86

Exercise 1M   *Fraction to a decimal II*

Part i

1 0.3	**3** 0.3	**5** 0.2	**7** 0.5
2 0.8	**4** 0.7	**6** 0.3	**8** 0.9

Part ii

1 0.67	**3** 0.86	**5** 0.89	**7** 0.91
2 0.17	**4** 0.44	**6** 0.36	**8** 0.42

Part iii

1 0.033	**3** 0.117	**5** 0.129	**7** 0.011
2 0.567	**4** 0.517	**6** 0.757	**8** 0.256

Exercise 1N   *Fraction to a decimal III*

Part i

1 $33.3 \Rightarrow 33$	**5** $18.7 \Rightarrow 19$	**9** $20.8 \Rightarrow 21$	**13** $46.8 \Rightarrow 47$
2 $83.3 \Rightarrow 83$	**6** $31.2 \Rightarrow 31$	**10** $45.8 \Rightarrow 46$	**14** $53.1 \Rightarrow 53$
3 $166.6 \Rightarrow 167$	**7** $14.4 \Rightarrow 14$	**11** $34.2 \Rightarrow 34$	**15** $27.7 \Rightarrow 28$
4 $183.3 \Rightarrow 183$	**8** $28.8 \Rightarrow 29$	**12** $42.8 \Rightarrow 43$	**16** $61.1 \Rightarrow 61$

Part ii

1 $1.66 \Rightarrow 1.7$	**5** $2.85 \Rightarrow 2.9$	**9** $3.12 \Rightarrow 3.1$	**13** $2.22 \Rightarrow 2.2$
2 $3.33 \Rightarrow 3.3$	**6** $3.57 \Rightarrow 3.6$	**10** $4.37 \Rightarrow 4.4$	**14** $5.55 \Rightarrow 5.6$
3 $5.83 \Rightarrow 5.8$	**7** $7.14 \Rightarrow 7.1$	**11** $6.87 \Rightarrow 6.9$	**15** $7.77 \Rightarrow 7.8$
4 $4.16 \Rightarrow 4.2$	**8** $9.28 \Rightarrow 9.3$	**12** $5.62 \Rightarrow 5.6$	**16** $9.44 \Rightarrow 9.4$

Exercise 10 *Mixed numbers and improper fractions*

Part i

1 $2\frac{1}{2}$	**5** $4\frac{5}{6}$	**9** $25\frac{1}{2}$	**13** $15\frac{5}{6}$	**17** $26\frac{3}{5}$
2 $3\frac{2}{3}$	**6** $5\frac{1}{7}$	**10** $21\frac{2}{3}$	**14** $14\frac{3}{7}$	**18** $23\frac{5}{6}$
3 $4\frac{1}{4}$	**7** $4\frac{5}{8}$	**11** $17\frac{3}{4}$	**15** $14\frac{1}{8}$	**19** $22\frac{3}{7}$
4 $4\frac{2}{5}$	**8** $5\frac{4}{9}$	**12** $17\frac{1}{5}$	**16** $13\frac{8}{9}$	**20** $18\frac{4}{9}$

Part ii

1 $\frac{3}{2}$	**5** $\frac{7}{2}$	**9** $\frac{67}{6}$	**13** $\frac{45}{2}$	**17** $\frac{185}{6}$
2 $\frac{4}{3}$	**6** $\frac{14}{3}$	**10** $\frac{93}{7}$	**14** $\frac{74}{3}$	**18** $\frac{228}{7}$
3 $\frac{7}{4}$	**7** $\frac{25}{4}$	**11** $\frac{133}{8}$	**15** $\frac{111}{4}$	**19** $\frac{283}{8}$
4 $\frac{13}{5}$	**8** $\frac{49}{5}$	**12** $\frac{155}{9}$	**16** $\frac{146}{5}$	**20** $\frac{347}{9}$

Exercise 1P *Multiplication of fractions*

1 $\frac{1}{5}$	**10** $\frac{3}{20}$	**19** $\frac{9}{10}$	**28** $\frac{3}{16}$
2 $\frac{5}{24}$	**11** $\frac{4}{9}$	**20** $\frac{9}{32}$	**29** $\frac{2}{15}$
3 $\frac{5}{9}$	**12** $\frac{1}{18}$	**21** 1	**30** $\frac{1}{5}$
4 $\frac{1}{6}$	**13** $\frac{11}{42}$	**22** $\frac{1}{135}$	**31** $\frac{27}{32}$
5 $1\frac{2}{3}$	**14** $\frac{3}{140}$	**23** $\frac{7}{18}$	**32** $\frac{1}{18}$
6 $\frac{3}{50}$	**15** $\frac{20}{21}$	**24** $\frac{5}{27}$	**33** $\frac{1}{360}$
7 $\frac{3}{5}$	**16** $\frac{12}{35}$	**25** $\frac{7}{15}$	**34** $\frac{7}{72}$
8 $\frac{9}{20}$	**17** $\frac{5}{28}$	**26** $\frac{7}{16}$	**35** $\frac{21}{160}$
9 $\frac{5}{6}$	**18** $\frac{1}{16}$	**27** $\frac{4}{27}$	**36** $\frac{121}{160}$

Chapter 2: Dosages of oral medications

Exercise 2A

1	2	**3**	$1\frac{1}{2}$	**5**	$1\frac{1}{2}$	**7**	$1\frac{1}{2}$	**9**	$2\frac{1}{2}$
2	$\frac{1}{2}$	**4**	2	**6**	$\frac{1}{2}$	**8**	$\frac{1}{2}$	**10**	$\frac{1}{2}$

Exercise 2B

1 **a** 2 mg + 2 mg (2 tabs)
   b 5 mg + 2 mg + 2 mg (3 tabs)
   c 10 mg + 2 mg (2 tabs)
   d 10 mg + 5 mg (2 tabs)

2 **a** 5 mg + 2 mg (2 tabs)
   b 5 mg + 2 mg + 2 mg (3 tabs)
   c 10 mg + 5 mg (2 tabs)
   d 10 mg + 10 mg (2 tabs)

3 **a** 120 mg + 80 mg (2 tabs); or 160 mg + 40 mg (2 tabs)
   b 120 mg + 120 mg (2 tabs); or 160 mg + 80 mg (2 tabs)
   c 160 mg + 120 mg (2 tabs)
   d 160 mg + 160 mg (2 tabs)

4 **a** 5 mg + 1 mg (2 tabs)
   b 5 mg + 2 mg + 1 mg (3 tabs)
   c 5 mg + 2 mg + 2 mg (3 tabs)
   d 5 mg + 5 mg + 1 mg (3 tabs)

5 **a** 40 mg + 20 mg (2 tabs)
   b 80 mg + 20 mg (2 tabs)
   c 80 mg + 80 mg + 40 mg (3 tabs)
   d 500 mg + 40 mg + 20 mg (3 tabs)

6 **a** 25 mg + 10 mg (2 tabs)
   b 50 mg + 10 mg (2 tabs)
   c 50 mg + 25 mg (2 tabs)
   d 100 mg + 10 mg + 10 mg (3 tabs)

Exercise 2C   *All answers are in milligrams (mg).*

1	**a** 20	**b** 30	**c** 50	**5**	**a** 40	**b** 100	**c** 160
2	**a** 6	**b** 10	**c** 14	**6**	**a** 500	**b** 1000	**c** 1500
3	**a** 80	**b** 200	**c** 400	**7**	**a** 50	**b** 150	**c** 250
4	**a** 500	**b** 750	**c** 1000	**8**	**a** 750	**b** 1250	**c** 1750

Exercise 2D   *All volumes are in millilitres (mL).*

1 20	**4** 7.5	**7** 7.5	**10** 24
2 4	**5** 6	**8** 20	**11** 32
3 2.5	**6** 25	**9** 7	

Exercise 2E

1 2 tablets	**3 a i** 10 mg	**ii** 20 mg	**b** 4 mL
2 2 tablets	**4 a i** 25 mg	**ii** 50 mg	**b** 8 mL

Chapter 2: Revision

1 2 [2A: 1I]

2 $\frac{1}{2}$ [2A: 1J]

3 $1\frac{1}{2}$ [2A: 1I]

4 **a** 2 mg + 1 mg (2 tabs)
   b 5 mg + 2 mg (2 tabs)
   c 10 mg + 2 mg + 1 mg (3 tabs)
   d 10 mg + 5 mg + 1 mg (3 tabs) [2B]

5 Shaken thoroughly

6 a 50 mg **b** 100 mg **c** 250 mg [2C: 1A]

7 a 750 mg **b** 1250 mg **c** 1750 mg [2C]

8 15 mL [2D: 1I, 1P]

9 25 mL [2D: 1I, 1P]

10 16 mL [2D: 1I, 1P]

11 15 mL [2D: 1I]

12 2.5 mL [2D: 1I, 1N]

Answers to chapter revisions

If you make an error in answering any of the questions in the chapter revision exercises, then refer back to the worked examples in the corresponding exercises and also to the relevant arithmetic skills [as listed in brackets after each answer].

Chapter 3: Drug dosages for injection

Exercise 3A

1	less than 1 mL	**5**	equal to 10 mL
2	more than 2 mL	**6**	less than 2 mL
3	less than 5 mL	**7**	more than 1 mL
4	more than 2 mL	**8**	more than 2 mL

Exercise 3B   *All answers are in millilitres (mL).*

1	0.8	**3**	0.9	**5**	1.3	**7**	1.5
2	1.4	**4**	2.5	**6**	1.7	**8**	3.0

Exercise 3C   *All answers are in millilitres (mL).*

1	5	**4**	4	**7**	1.3
2	3.2	**5**	0.8	**8**	1.6
3	0.5	**6**	0.2	**9**	0.55

Exercise 3D   *All answers are in millilitres (mL).*

1	1.2	**4**	1.6	**7**	0.6
2	1.5	**5**	4	**8**	0.6
3	2.5	**6**	1.5	**9**	3.75 $\Rightarrow$ 3.8

Exercise 3E   *All answers are in millilitres (mL).*

1	6.7	**4**	0.67	**7**	1.4
2	1.3	**5**	0.88	**8**	1.8
3	0.83	**6**	0.43	**9**	1.3

Exercise 3F   *All answers are in millilitres (mL).*

1	0.8	**6**	1.6	**11**	4	**16**	3.8
2	0.28	**7**	1.2	**12**	2.4	**17**	1.3
3	12.5	**8**	0.8	**13**	1.8	**18**	0.75
4	0.6	**9**	3	**14**	4	**19**	6
5	0.35	**10**	2.5	**15**	0.75	**20**	1.3

Exercise 3G *All answers are in millilitres (mL).*

| **1** 4 | **2** 6 | **3** 0.5 | **4** 3.5 |

Exercise 3H

1 a $\frac{1}{100}$ mL = 0.01 mL   **b** A 0.20 mL   B 0.38 mL   C 0.73 mL
D 0.55 mL

2 a 2 units   **b** A 40 units   B 4 units   C 75 units   D 65 units

3 a $\frac{1}{10}$ mL = 0.1 mL   **b** A 1.2 mL   B 2.15 mL   C 2.6 mL

4 a $\frac{1}{5}$ mL = 0.2 mL   **b** A 2.2 mL   B 4.5 mL   C 3.9 mL

Chapter 3: Revision

All volumes are in millilitres (mL). Volumes more than 1 mL are rounded off to one decimal place; volumes less than 1 mL are given to two decimal places.

1 less than 1 mL [3A]
2 1.4 [3B, 3C, 3D: 1B, 1H, 1P]
3 2.4 [3B, 3C, 3D: 1G, 1H, 1N, 1P]
4 7.5 [3B, 3C, 3D: 1I, 1N, 1P]
5 1.1 [3B, 3C, 3D: 1I, 1L, 1P]
6 1.5 [3B, 3C, 3D: 1G, 1N, 1P]
7 9.0 [3B, 3C, 3D: 1C, 1H, 1P]
8 0.9 [3B, 3C, 3D: 1J, 1L, 1P]
9 6.33 $\Rightarrow$ 6.3 [3E, 3F: 1H, 1K, 1M, 1P]
10 0.666 $\Rightarrow$ 0.67 [3E, 3F: 1G, 1K, 1M]

Chapter 4: Intravenous infusion

Exercise 4A

1 **a** 84 mL   **b** 336 mL   **c** 504 mL
2 **a** 375 mL   **b** 625 mL   **c** 1500 mL
3 **a** 90 mL   **b** 150 mL   **c** 720 mL
4 20 hours
5 $12\frac{1}{2}$ hours = 12 h 30 min
6 $6\frac{2}{3}$ hours = 6 h 40 min
7 $\frac{2}{3}$ h = 40 min

Exercise 4B   *All answers are in mL/h.*

1 125	**6** 62.5 $\Rightarrow$ 63
2 41.6 $\Rightarrow$ 42	**7** 62.5 $\Rightarrow$ 63
3 71.4 $\Rightarrow$ 71	**8** 41.6 $\Rightarrow$ 42
4 133.3 $\Rightarrow$ 133	**9** 160
5 166.6 $\Rightarrow$ 167	**10** 200

Exercise 4C   *All answers are in mL/h.*

1 120	**5** 102.8 $\Rightarrow$ 103
2 144	**6** 106.6 $\Rightarrow$ 107
3 200	**7** 112.5 $\Rightarrow$ 113
4 100	**8** 168

Exercise 4D   *All answers are in drops/min.*

1 25	**6** 50
2 20.8 $\Rightarrow$ 21	**7** 120
3 13.8 $\Rightarrow$ 14	**8** 40
4 27.7 $\Rightarrow$ 28	**9** 24
5 33.3 $\Rightarrow$ 33	

Exercise 4E   *All answers are in drops/min.*

1 $20.8 \Rightarrow 21$	**5** $29.1 \Rightarrow 29$
2 $41.6 \Rightarrow 42$	**6** 40
3 $41.6 \Rightarrow 42$	**7** $34.2 \Rightarrow 34$
4 50	**8** 35

Exercise 4F

1 1800 mL

2 Running time = $13\frac{1}{3}$ h = 13 h 20 min
Finishing time = 0800 h + 13 h 20 min = 2120 hours

3 Running time = 20 h
Finishing time = 2100 h Monday + 20 h = 1700 hours Tuesday

4 6 h + 7 h = 13 hours

5 Total running time = 5 h + $2\frac{1}{2}$ h = $7\frac{1}{2}$ h = 7 h 30 min
Finishing time = 0800 h + 7 h 30 min = 1530 hours

6 Total running time = 10 h + 8 h = 18 h
Finishing time = 0430 h + 18 h = 2230 hours

7 110 mL/h

8 55 mL/h

Exercise 4G

1 a 0.7 mg/mL   **b i** 7 mg   **ii** 10.5 mg   **iii** 17.5 mg   **iv** 28 mg
   c i $12.8 \Rightarrow 13$ mL/h   **ii** $17.1 \Rightarrow 17$ mL/h   **iii** $28.5 \Rightarrow 29$ mL/h
   iv $35.7 \Rightarrow 36$ mL/h

2 a 0.1 mg/mL   **b i** 1 mg   **ii** 1.5 mg   **iii** 2 mg   **iv** 4 mg
   c i 15 mL/h   **ii** 25 mL/h   **iii** 30 mL/h   **iv** 35 mL/h

3 a 10 mcg/mL [*Note* mcg]   **b** 10 mcg   **c** 60 mcg

Exercise 4H   *All answers are in kilojoules.*

1 800	**5** 0 (no carbohydrate)
2 2000	**6** 480
3 1600	**7** 0 (no carbohydrate)
4 2000	**8** 400

Chapter 4: Revision

1 a 110 mL   **b** 275 mL   **c** 605 mL [4A]

2 $8\frac{1}{3}$ h = 8 h 20 min   [4A: 1C, 1I, 1O]

3 75 mL/h   [4B: 1C, 1I]

4 90.9 $\Rightarrow$ 91 mL/h   [4B: 1C, 1I, 1K, 1N]

5 133.3 $\Rightarrow$ 133 mL/h   [4C: 1I, 1K, 1N, 1P]

6 50 drops/min   [4D: 1I, 1P]

7 27.7 $\Rightarrow$ 28 drops/min   [4E: 1G, 1K, 1N, 1P]

8 50 drops/min   [4D: 1C, 1G, 1I, 1P]

9 20.8 $\Rightarrow$ 21 drops/min   [4D: 1C, 1G, 1I, 1K, 1N, 1P]

10 1620 mL   [4F]

11 Running time = $12\frac{1}{2}$ h = 12 h 30 min

Finishing time = 0700 h + 12 h 30 min = 1930 hours

[4F: 1C, 1I, 1O]

12 6 h + 11 h = 17 h   [4F: 1C, 1I]

13 Total running time = 8 h + 11 h = 19 h

Finishing time = 0300 h + 19 h = 2200 hours   [4F: 1C, 1I]

14 115 mL/h   [4F: 1C, 1I, 1N]

15 a 0.5 mg/mL   **b** 2.5 mg/h   **c** 7 mL/h   [4G: 1B, 1E, 1G, 1J]

16 a 10 mcg/mL   **b** 10 mcg   **c** 50 mcg   [4G: 1E, 1I]

17 1200 kJ   [4H: 1C, 1H]

Chapter 5: Paediatric dosages

Exercise 5A *All answers are in milligrams (mg).*

1	120	**4**	250	**7**	900
2	150	**5**	200	**8**	240
3	90	**6**	225	**9**	540

Exercise 5B *All answers are in millilitres (mL).*

1	0.4	**7**	0.4	**13**	0.25	**19**	0.45
2	0.4	**8**	0.75	**14**	7.2	**20**	0.8
3	0.8	**9**	0.48	**15**	0.65	**21**	1.5
4	0.75	**10**	1.2	**16**	1.5	**22**	2.5
5	0.5	**11**	1.2	**17**	1.0		
6	0.72	**12**	0.3	**18**	0.8		

Exercise 5C *All answers are in millilitres (mL).*

1	3.5	**5**	2.5	**9**	$11.25 \Rightarrow 11.3$	**13**	4.0
2	12.5	**6**	4	**10**	$2.25 \Rightarrow 2.3$		
3	12.5	**7**	8	**11**	0.6		
4	7	**8**	14	**12**	0.5		

Exercise 5D *All answers are in millilitres (mL).*

1 a 1.2 **b** 0.9 **c** 0.6   **3 a** 0.4 **b** 0.6 **c** 0.8
2 a 1.5 **b** 1.2 **c** 0.75 **d** 0.6 **4 a** 0.88 **b** $1.32 \Rightarrow 1.3$ **c** $1.54 \Rightarrow 1.5$

Exercise 5E *All answers are in m^2.*

1	**a** 0.35	**4**	**a** 0.57	**7**	**a** 0.51	**9**	**a** 0.45
	b 0.40		**b** 0.64		**b** 0.53		**b** 0.45
2	**a** 0.43	**5**	**a** 0.31	**8**	**a** 0.59	**10**	**a** 0.57
	b 0.48		**b** 0.32		**b** 0.61		**b** 0.57
3	**a** 0.51	**6**	**a** 0.43				
	b 0.57		**b** 0.45				

Exercise 5F *All answers are in mL.*

1	1.2	**2**	1.8	**3**	2.7	**4**	3.9	**5**	0.96	**6**	28.5

Chapter 5: Revision

1 275 mg   [5A]
2 285 mg   [5A]
3 180 mg   [5A]
4 0.6 mL   [5B: 1G, 1L, 1P]
5 0.96 mL   [5B: 1B, 1C, 1H, 1L]
6 0.6 mL   [5B: 1E, 1G, 1L]
7 7.5 mL   [5C: 1I, 1N, 1P]
8 0.72 mL   [5C: 1J, 1L]
9 12 mL   [5C: 1I, 1P]
10 **a** 1.6 mL   **b** 0.8 mL   **c** 0.64 mL   [5D: 1H, 1I, 1L]
11 **a** 0.30 mL   **b** 0.32 mL   **c** 0.70 mL   **d** 0.72 mL   [5D: 1G, 1L]
12 0.68 m^2 [5E]
13 0.74 m^2 [5E]
14 0.82 m^2 [5E]
15 0.90 m^2 [5E]
16 1.6 mL   [5F: 1B, 1E, 1J, 1N, 1P]
17 10.5 mL   [5F: 1B, 1E, 1J, 1N, 1P]

Chapter 6: Summary exercises

Summary exercise I

1 $1\frac{1}{2}$ tablets   [2A]

2 **a** 2 mg + 2 mg (2 tabs)   **b** 5 mg + 2 mg + 1 mg (3 tabs)
   c 10 mg + 2 mg (2 tabs)   [2B]

3 **a** 360 mg   **b** 600 mg   **c** 960 mg   [2C]

4 14.4 mL   [2D]

5 more than 5 mL   [3A]

6 4.5 mL   [3B]

7 1.33 $\Rightarrow$ 1.3 mL   [3C]

8 **a** 75 mL   **b** 125 mL   **c** 300 mL   [4A]

9 83.3 $\Rightarrow$ 83 mL/h   [4B]

10 168 mL/h   [4C]

11 29.1 $\Rightarrow$ 29 drops/min   [4D]

12 27.7 $\Rightarrow$ 28 drops/min   [4E]

13 5 h + $7\frac{1}{2}$ h = $12\frac{1}{2}$ h = 12 h 30 min   [4F]

14 **a** 0.8 mg/mL   **b** 12 mg/h   **c** 25 mL/h   [4G]

15 800 kJ   [4H]

16 225 mg/dose   [5A]

17 0.7 mL   [5B]

18 0.35 mL   [5C]

19 2.5 mL   [5C]

20 **a** 0.583 $\Rightarrow$ 0.58 mL   **b** 0.875 $\Rightarrow$ 0.88 mL
   c 1.16 $\Rightarrow$ 1.2 mL   [5D]

21 0.43 m^2 [5E]

22 0.99 mL   [5F]

Answers to Summary exercise I

*If you make an error in answering any of the questions in this
summary exercise, then refer back to the corresponding exercises in
Chapters 2–5 [as given in brackets after each answer above].*

Summary exercise II

1 $\frac{1}{2}$ tablet [2A]
2 **a** 50 mg + 10 mg (2 tabs)   **b** 50 mg + 25 mg + 10 mg (3 tabs)
   c 100 mg + 10 mg (2 tabs)   [2B]
3 **a** 60 mg **b** 120 mg **c** 140 mg [2C]
4 18 mL [2D]
5 less than 3 mL [3A]
6 0.9 mL [3B]
7 $12\frac{1}{2}$ hours = 12 h 30 min [4A]
8 55.5 $\Rightarrow$ 56 mL/h [4B]
9 200 mL/h [4C]
10 24 drops/min [4D]
11 30 drops/min [4E]
12 Running time = 12 h 30 min
   Finishing time = 2200 h Wednesday + 12 h 30 min = 1030
   hours Thursday [4F]
13 12 h + 5 h = 17 hours [4F]
14 **a** 10 mcg/mL **b** 10 mcg/dose **c** 40 mcg [4G]
15 1280 kJ [4H]
16 160 mg/dose [5A]
17 1.4 mL [5B]
18 6 mL [5B]
19 7 mL [5C]
20 **a** 0.25 mL **b** 0.45 mL **c** 0.6 mL [5D]
21 0.58 m^2 [5E]
22 0.9 mL [5F]

Answers to Summary exercise II

*If you make an error in answering any of the questions in this
summary exercise, then refer back to the corresponding exercises in
Chapters 2–5 [as given in brackets after each answer above].*

Index

NOTE: Individual types of drugs have not been indexed, only drug formulations, e.g. tablets, oral medications, etc.